This book belongs to:

_____

IF YOU ENJOYED THIS BOOK, I WOULD GREATLY APPRECIATE IF YOU COULD TAKE A
MOMENT TO LEAVE A REVIEW. THANK YOU FOR YOUR SUPPORT!

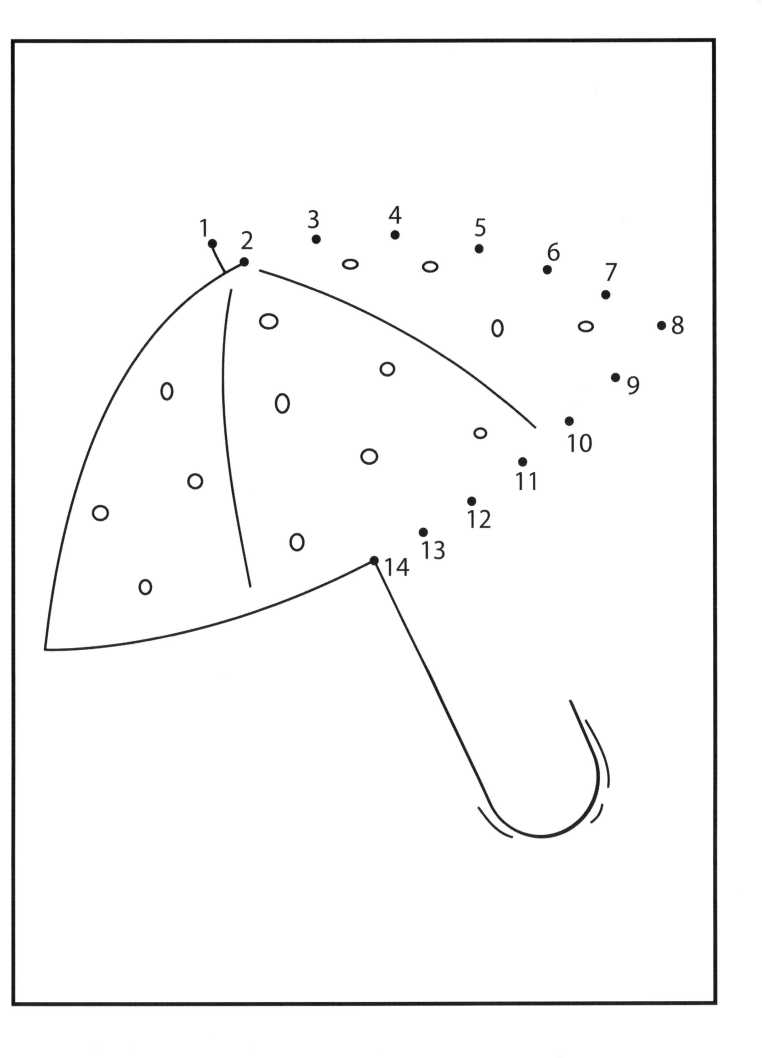

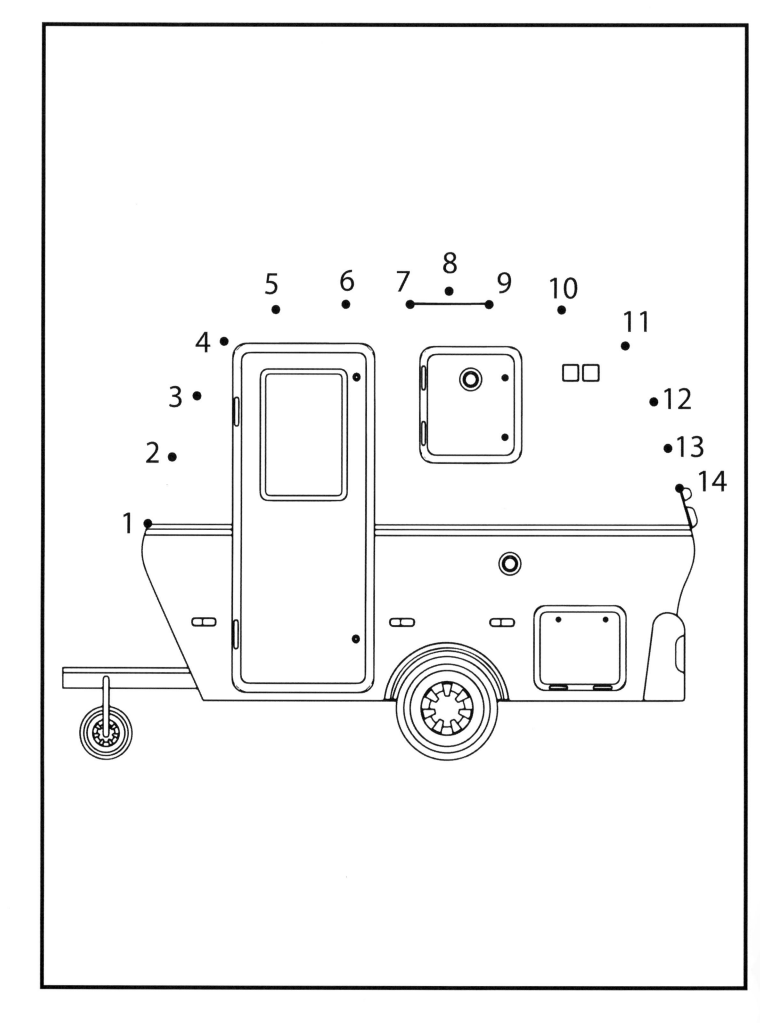

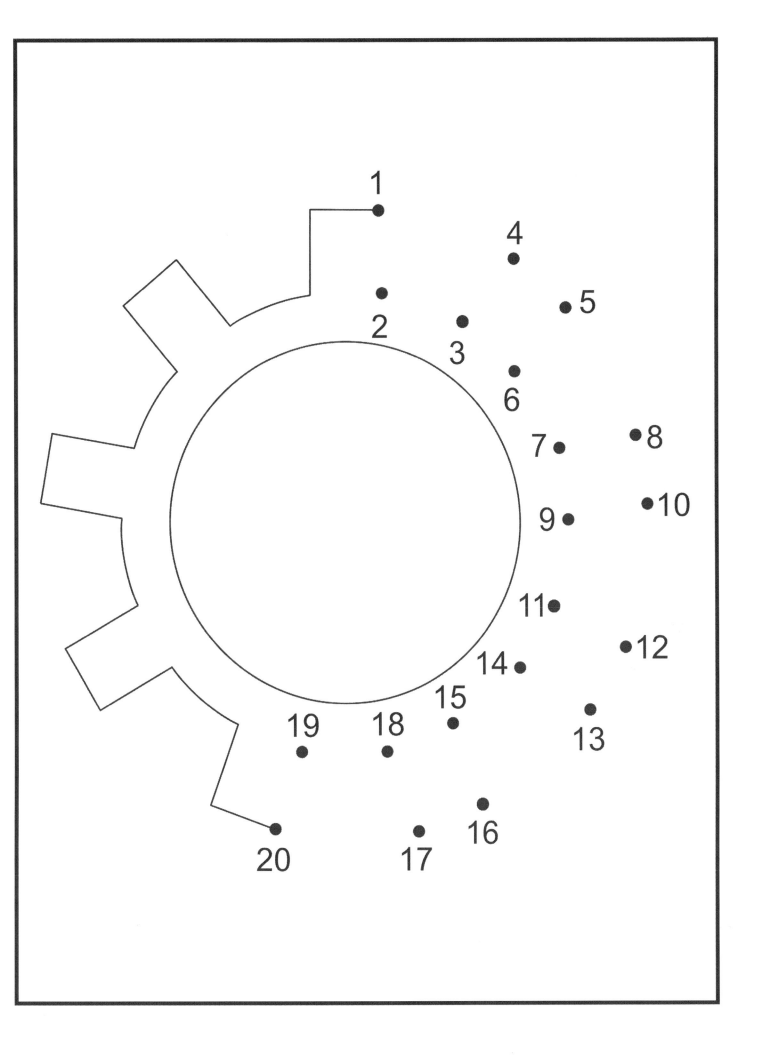

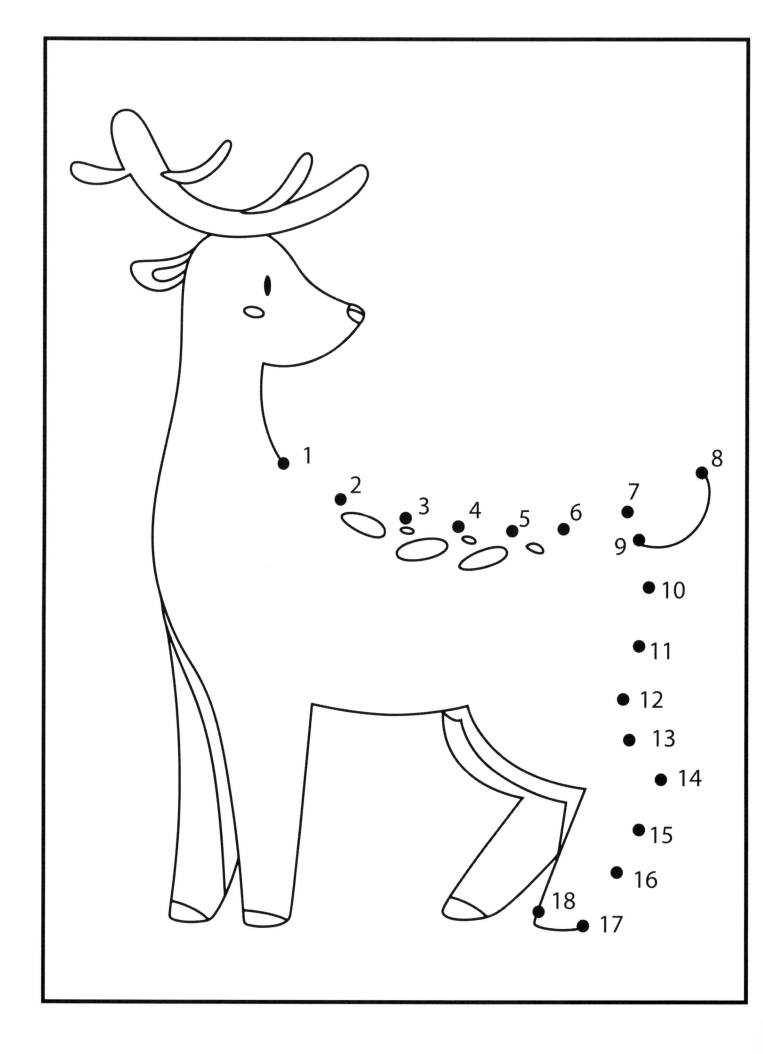

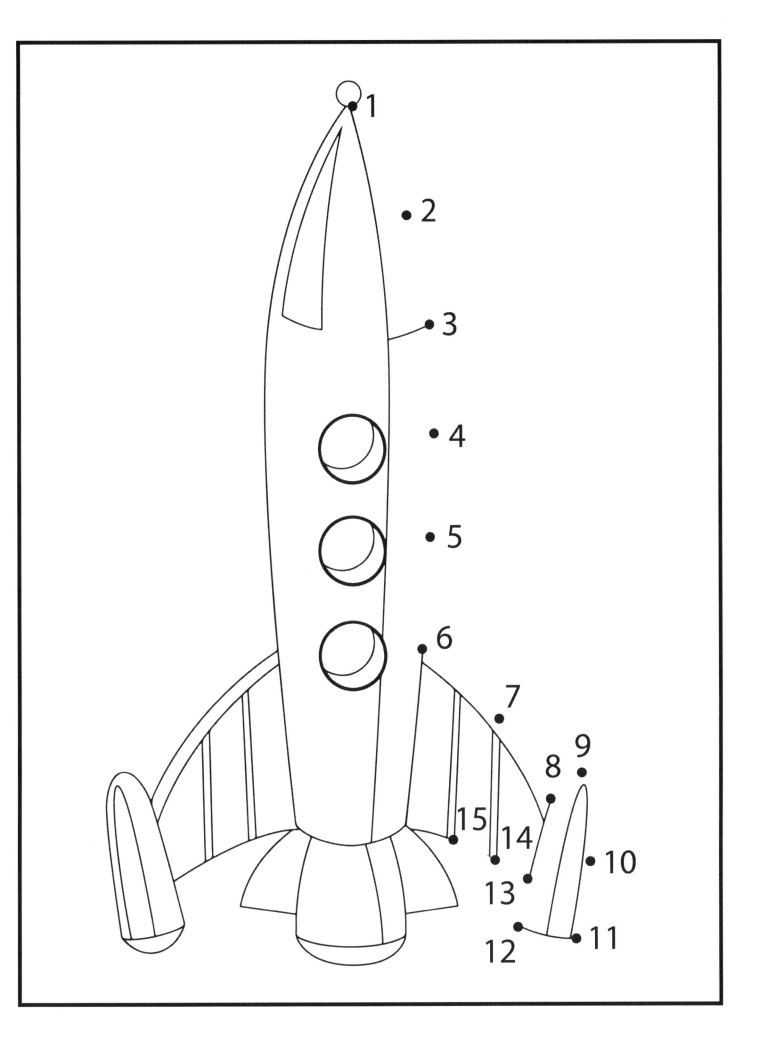

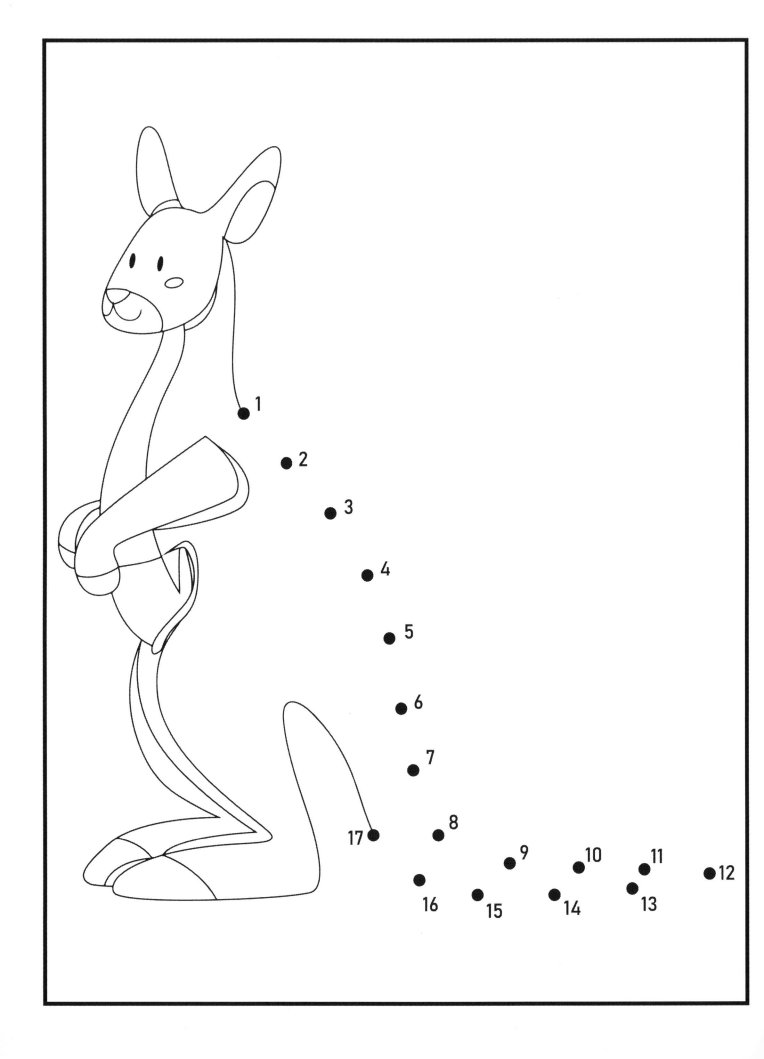

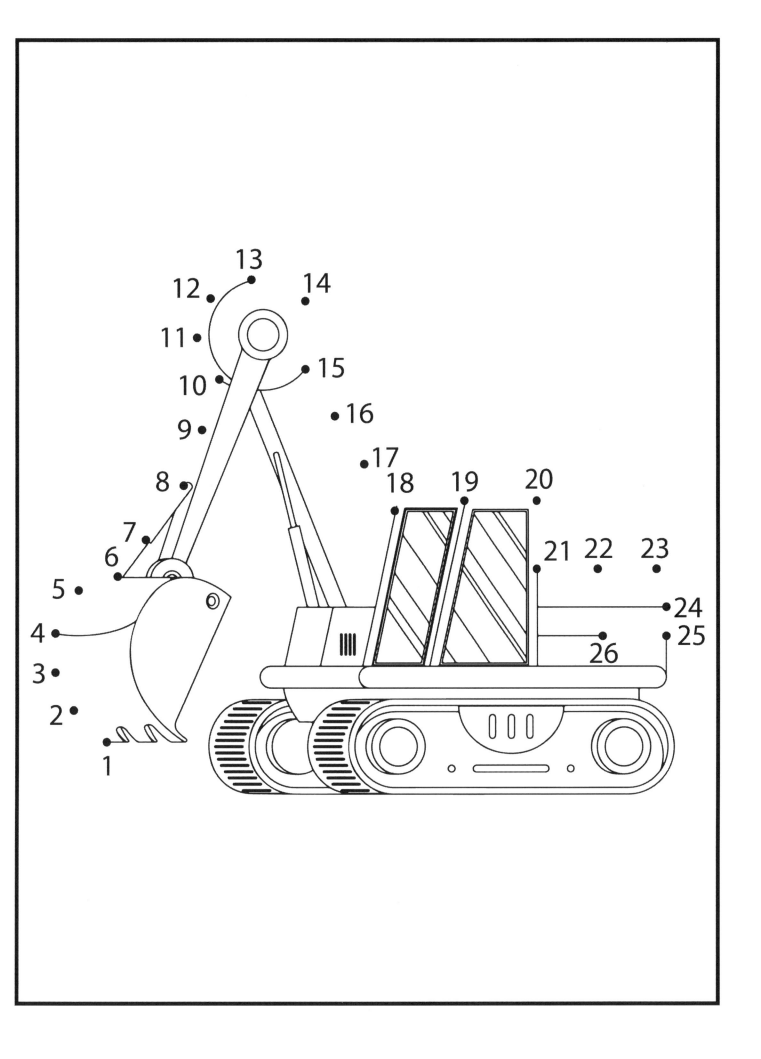

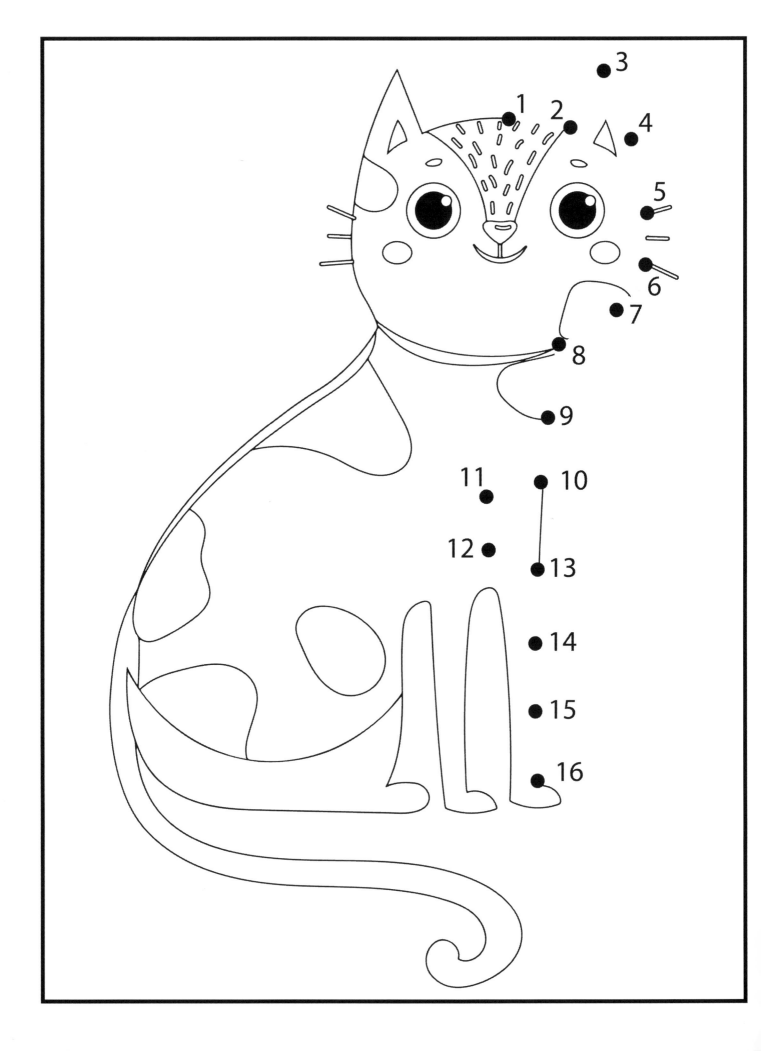

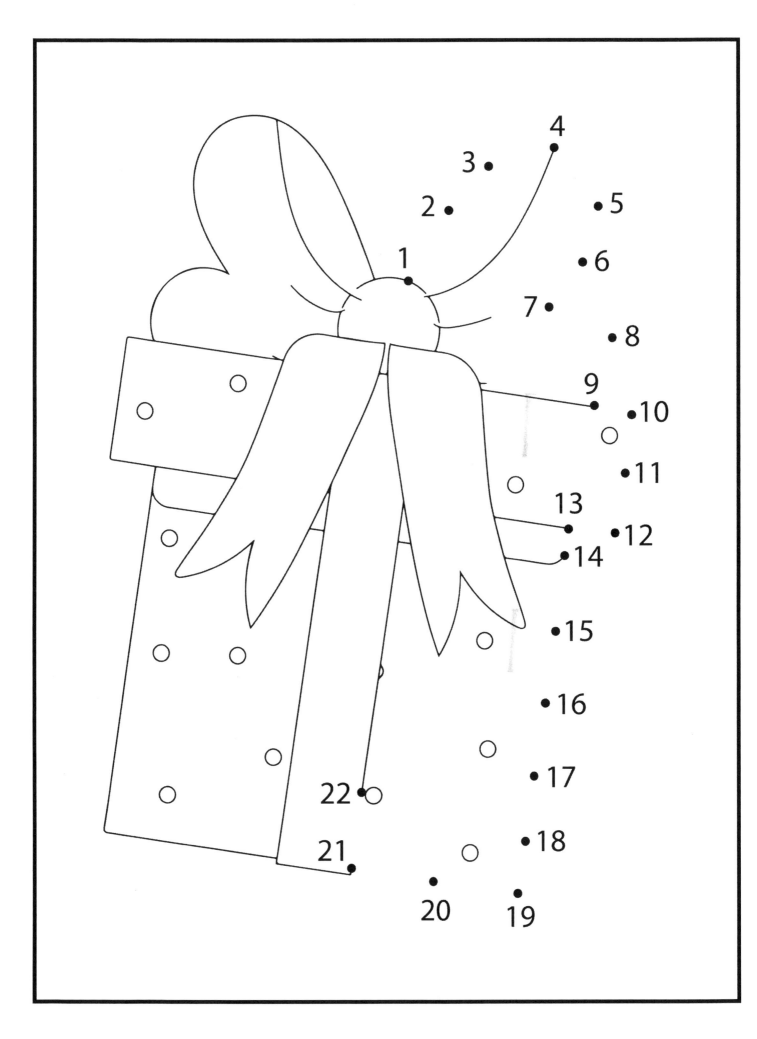

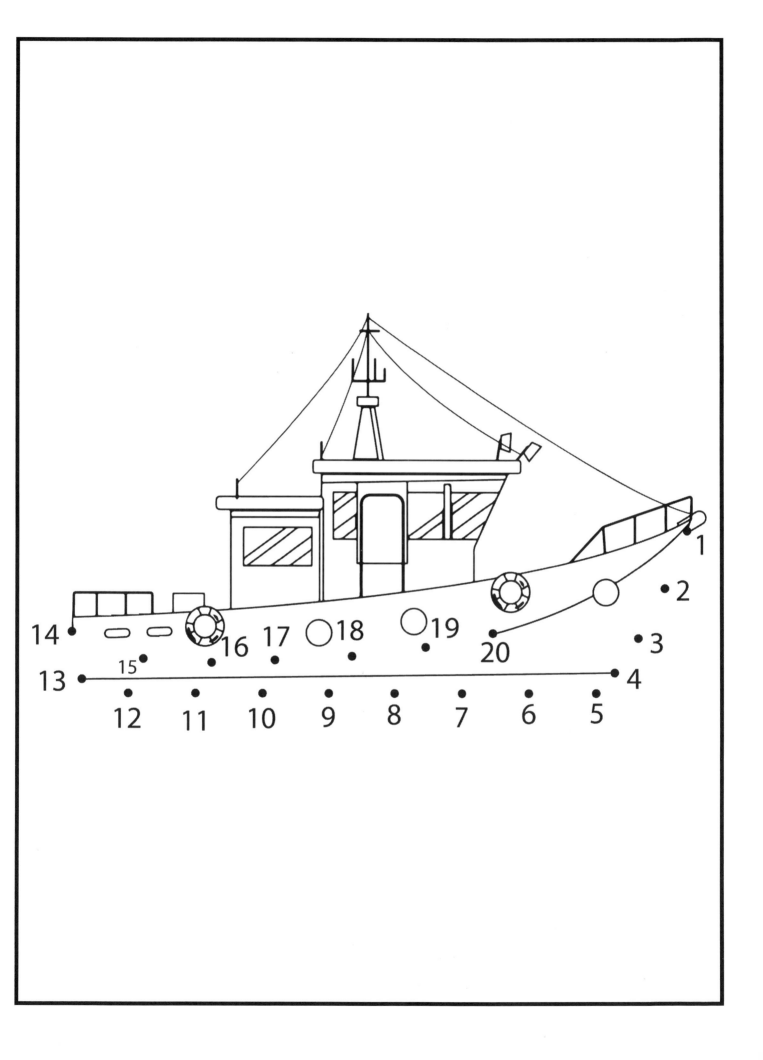

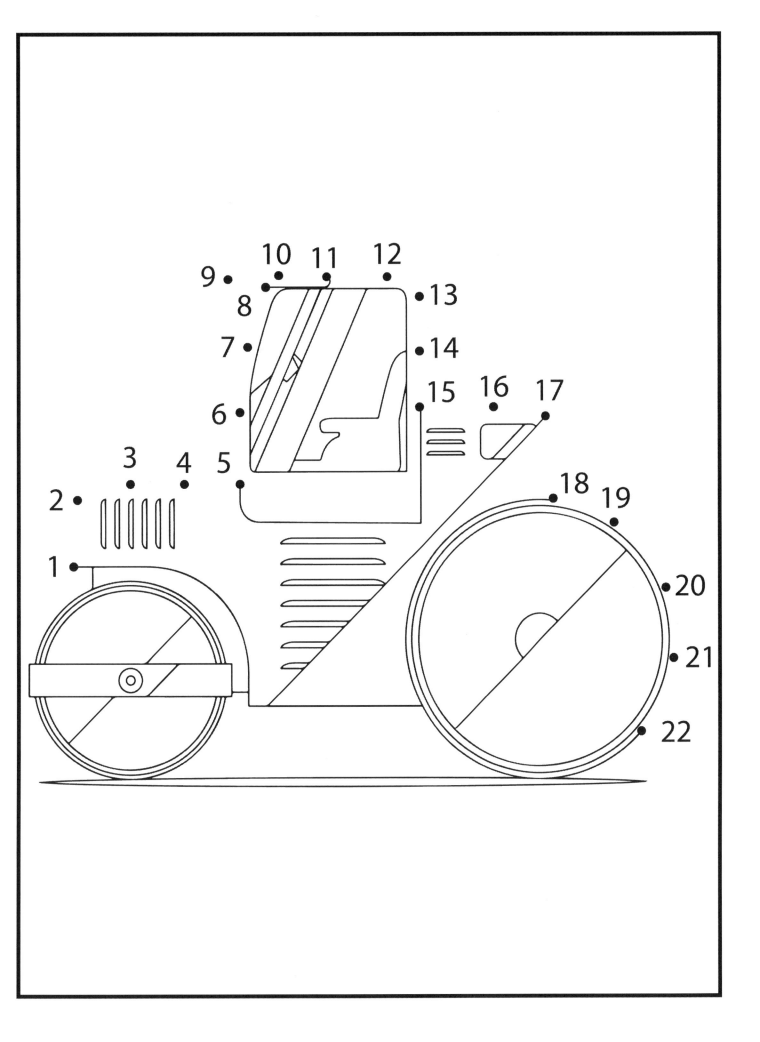

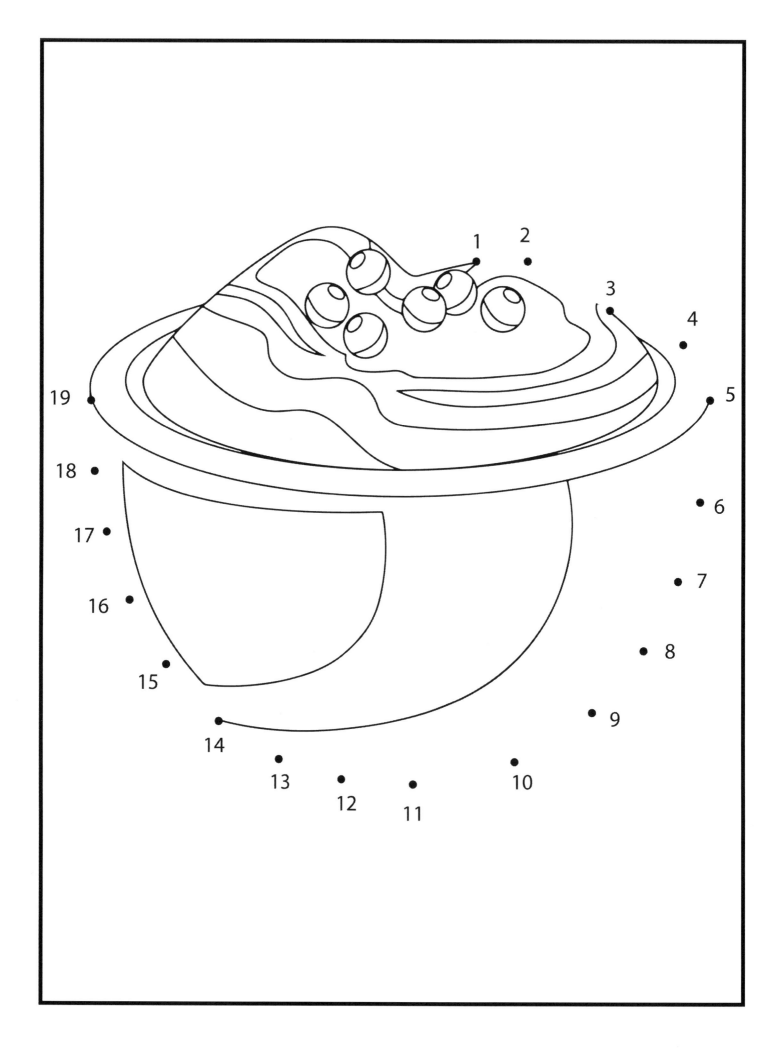

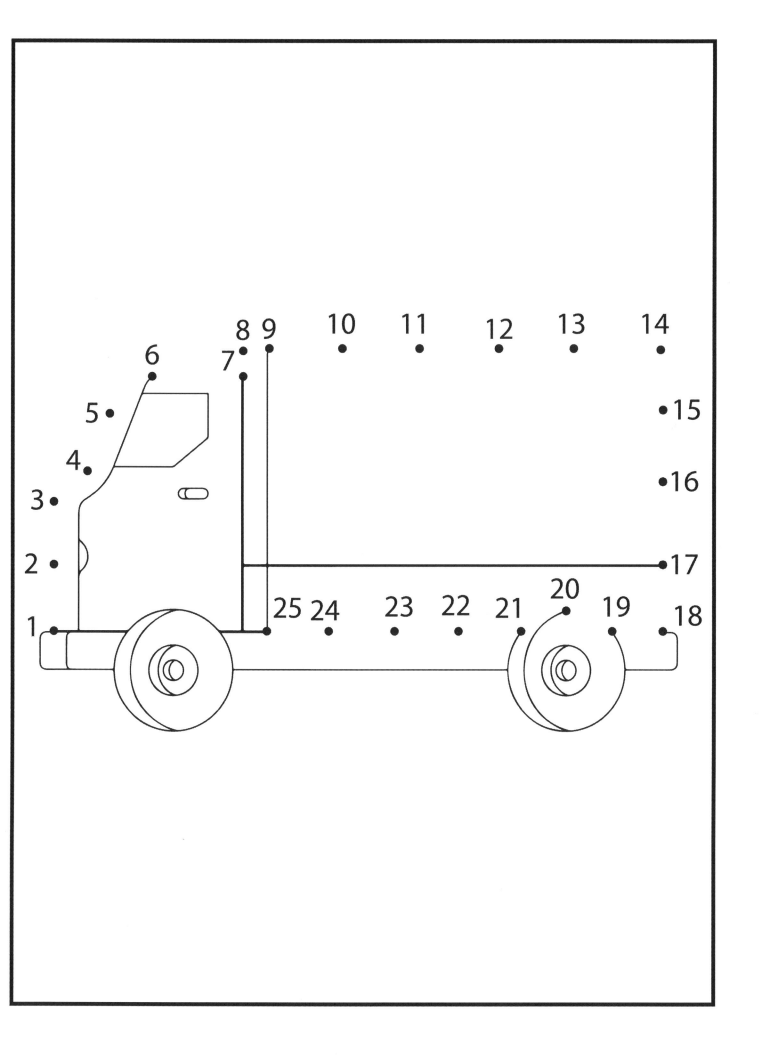

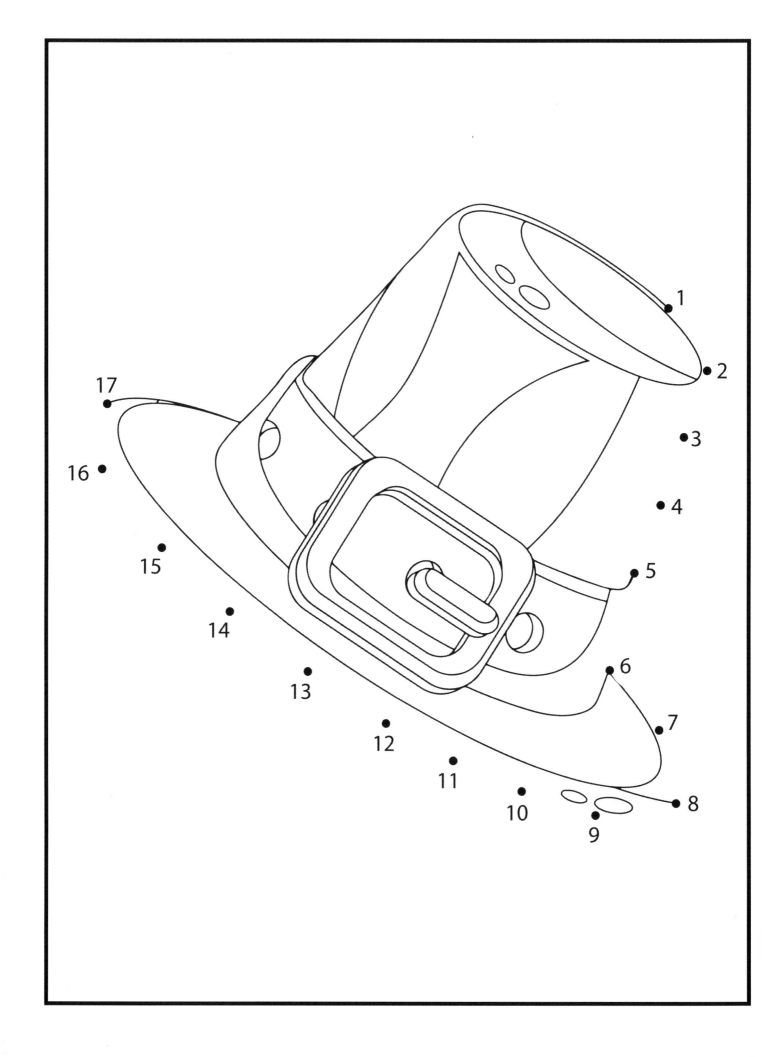

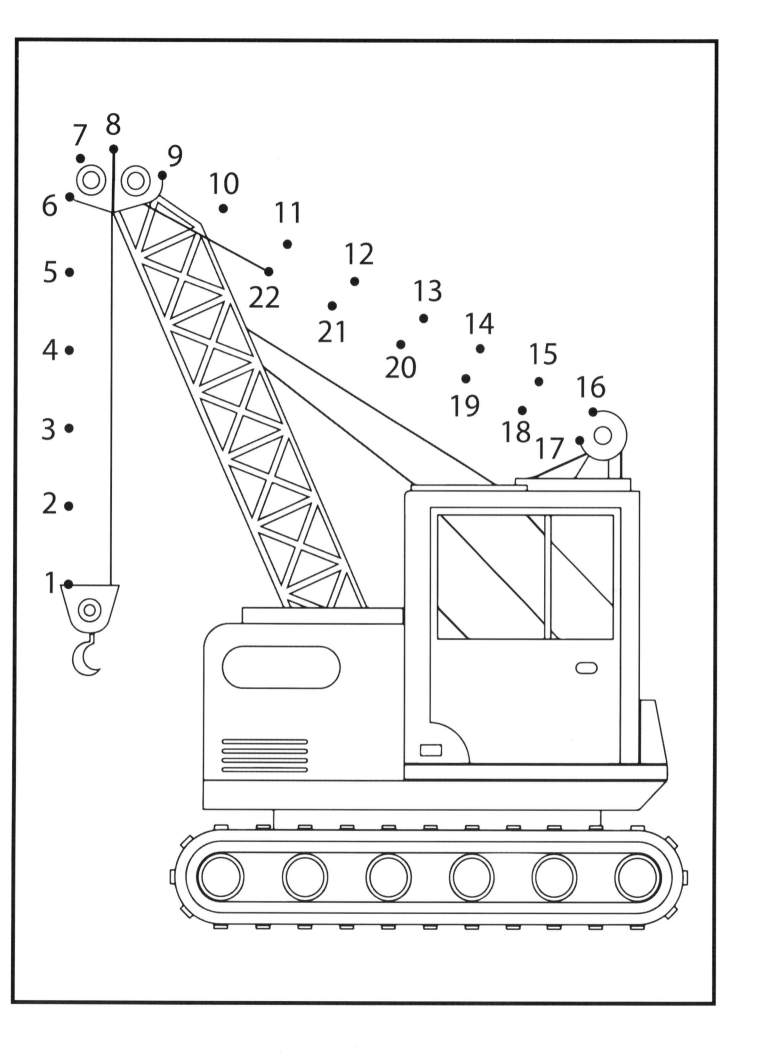

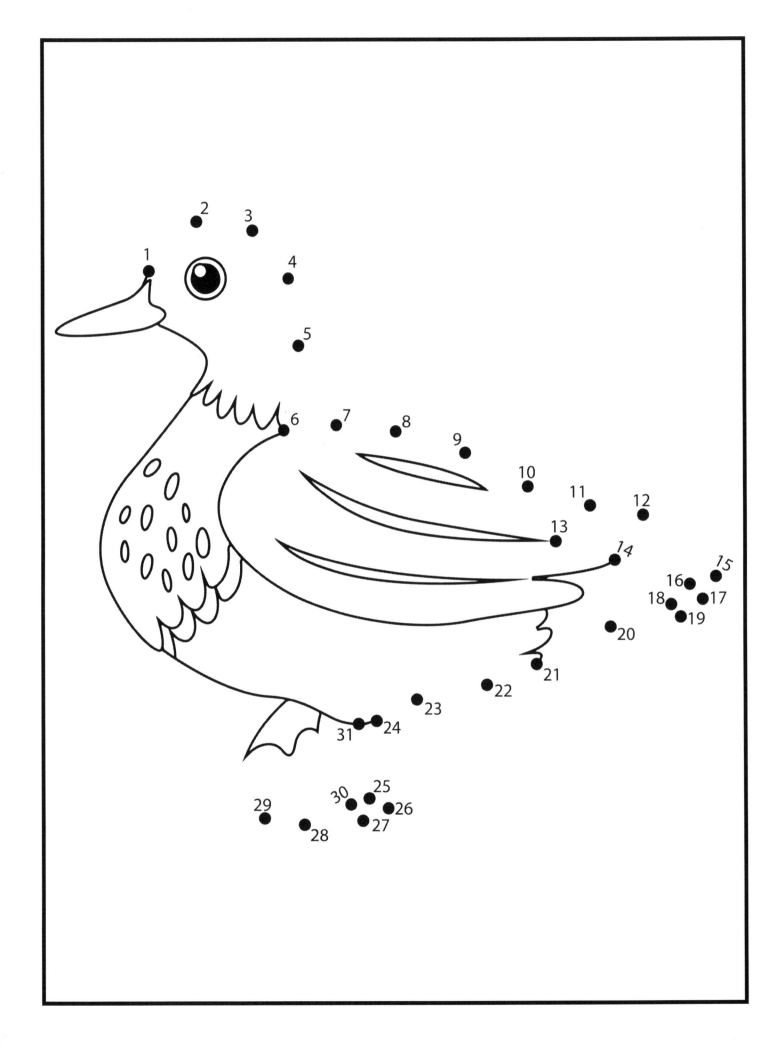

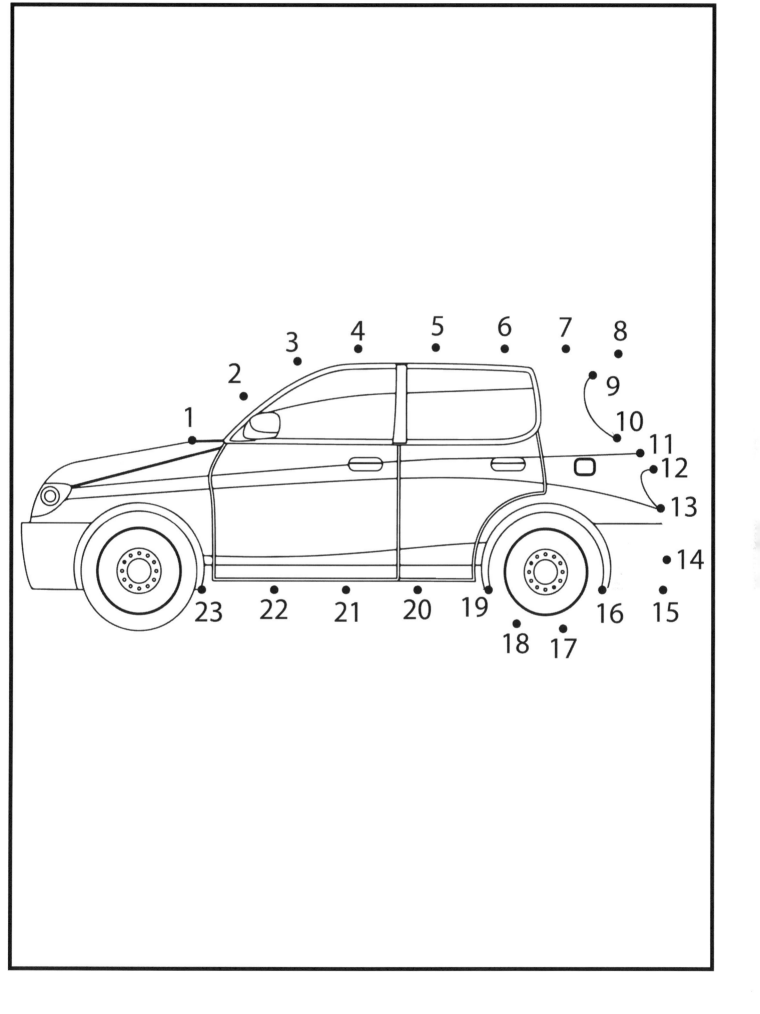

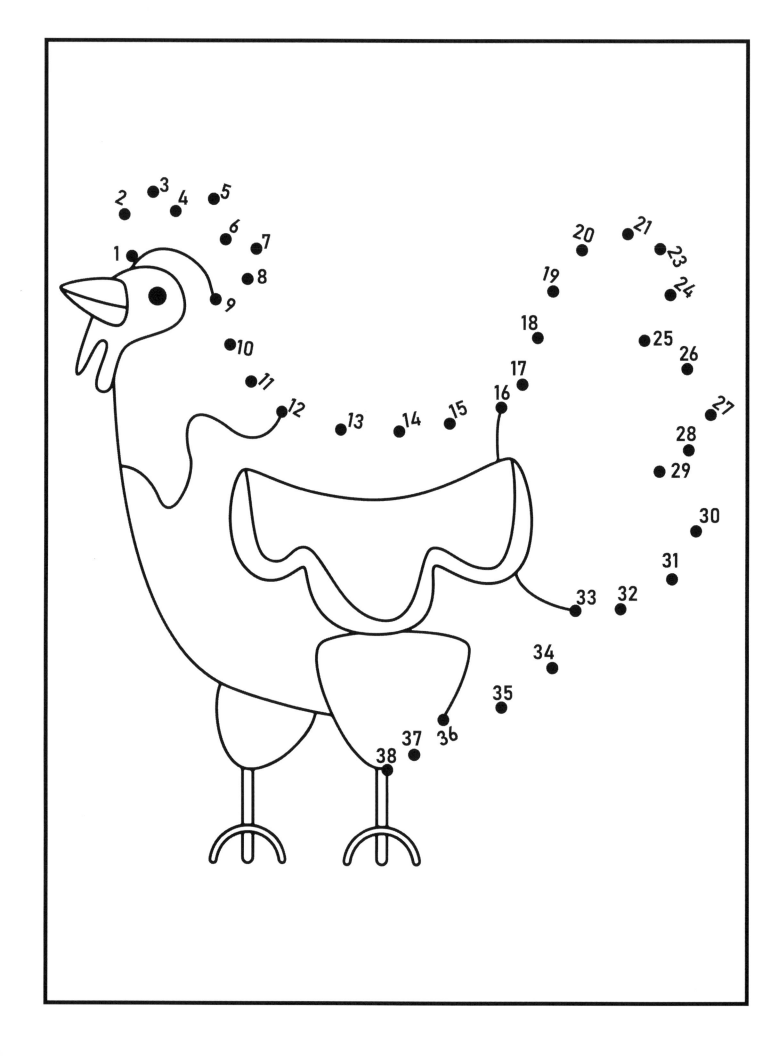

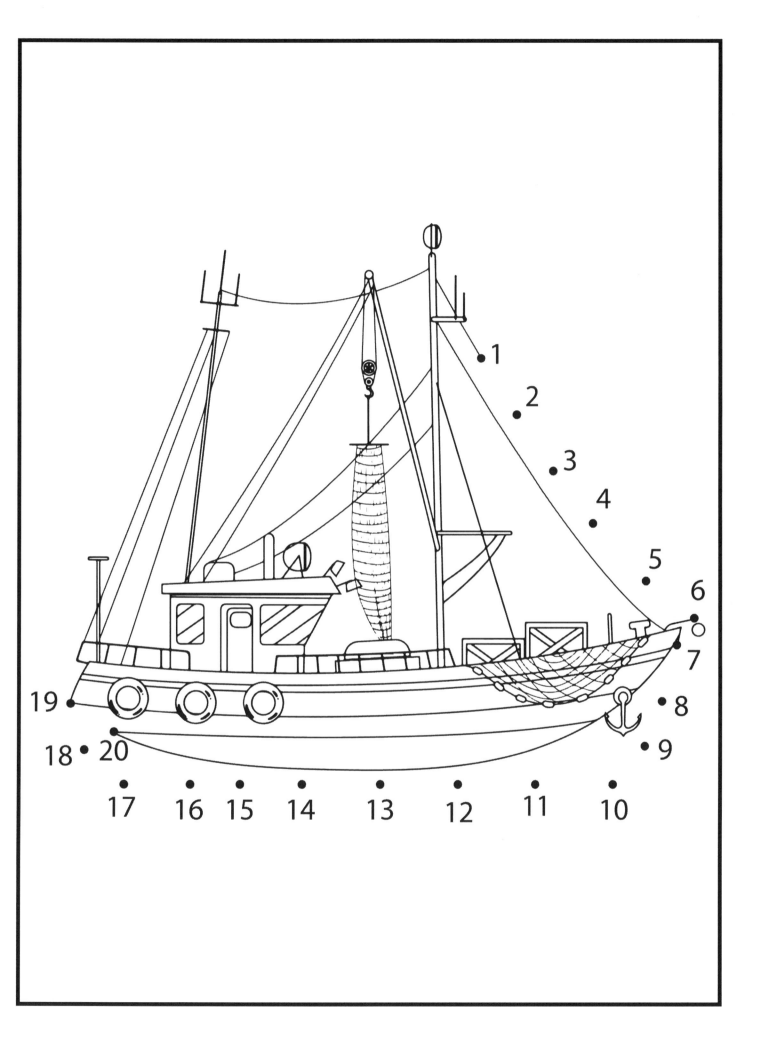

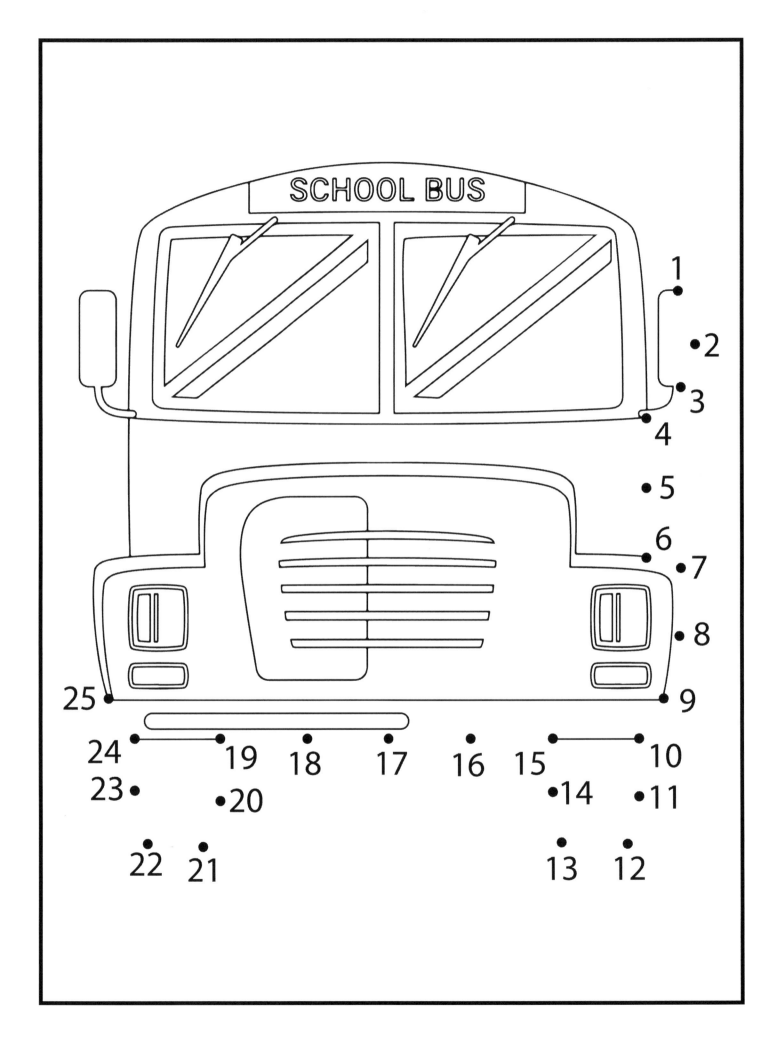

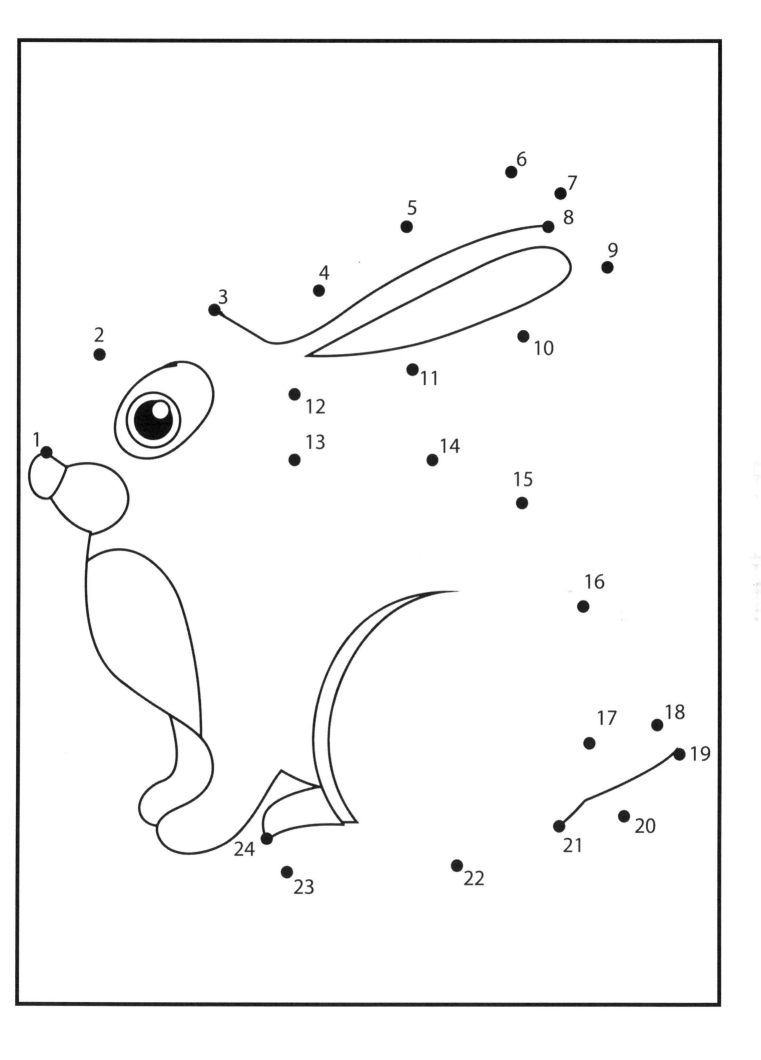

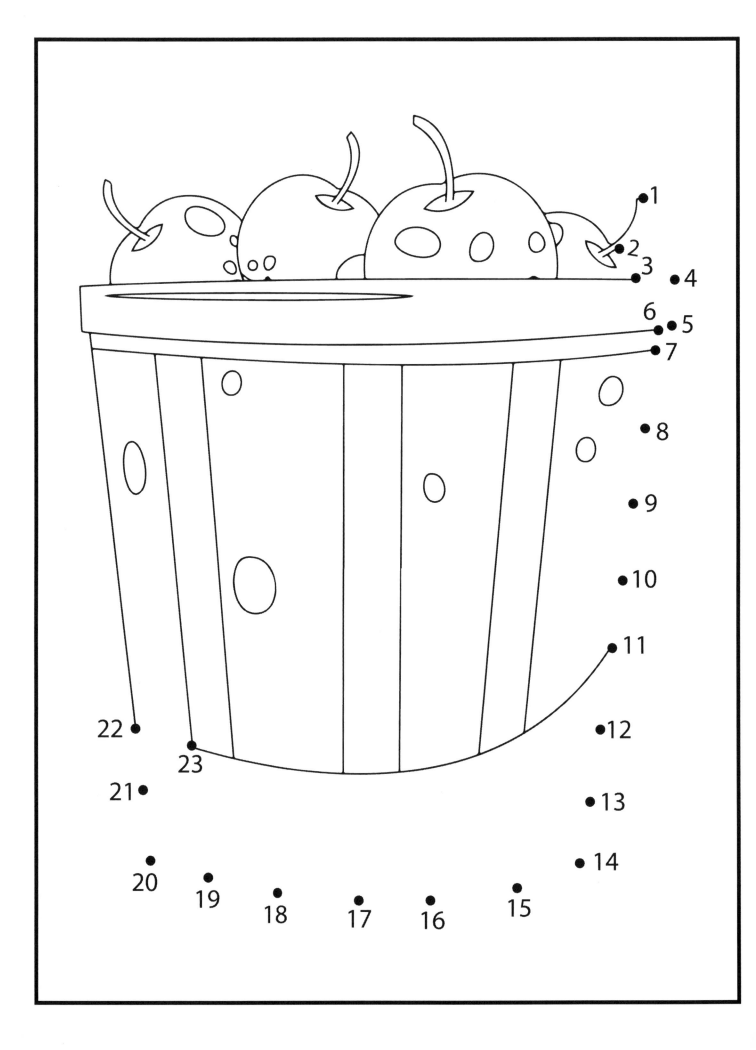

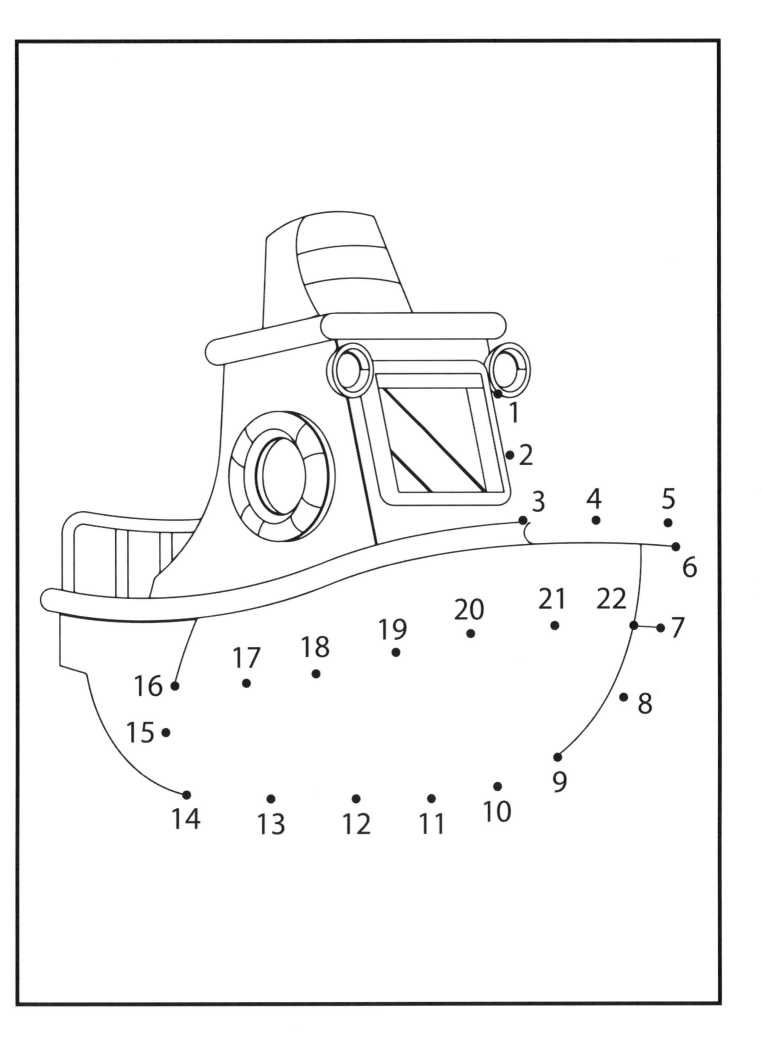

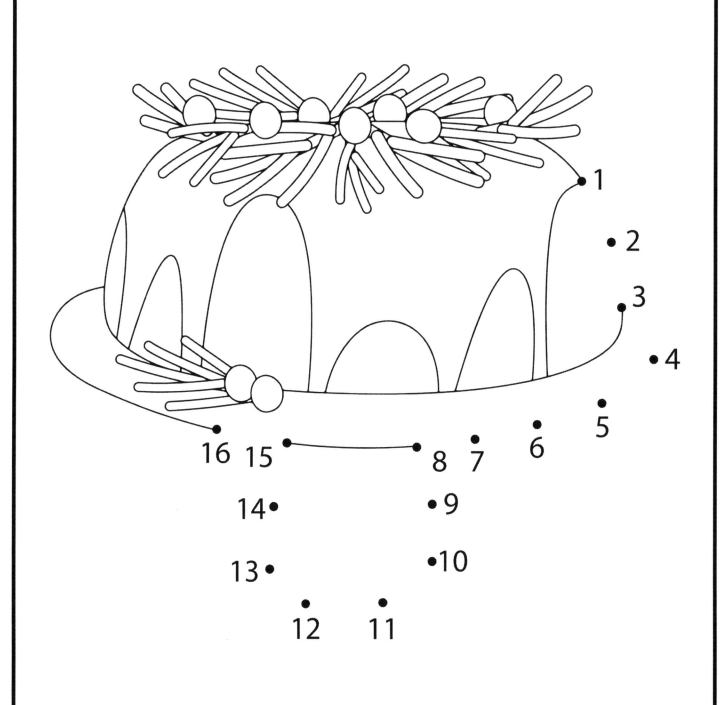

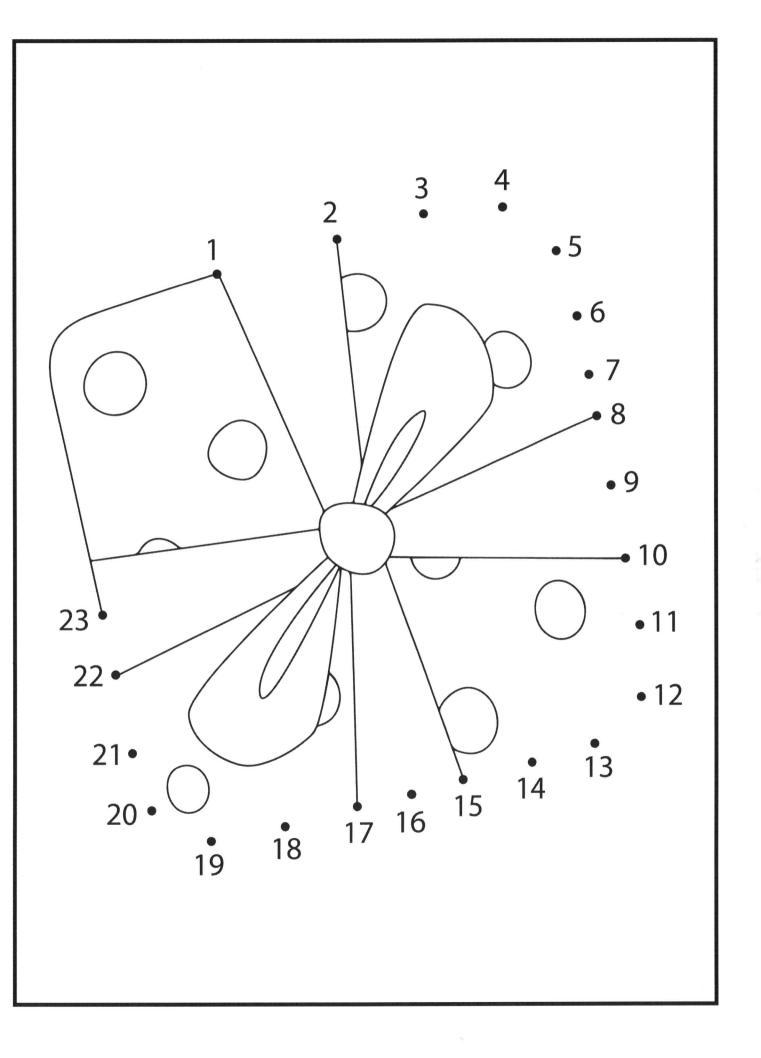

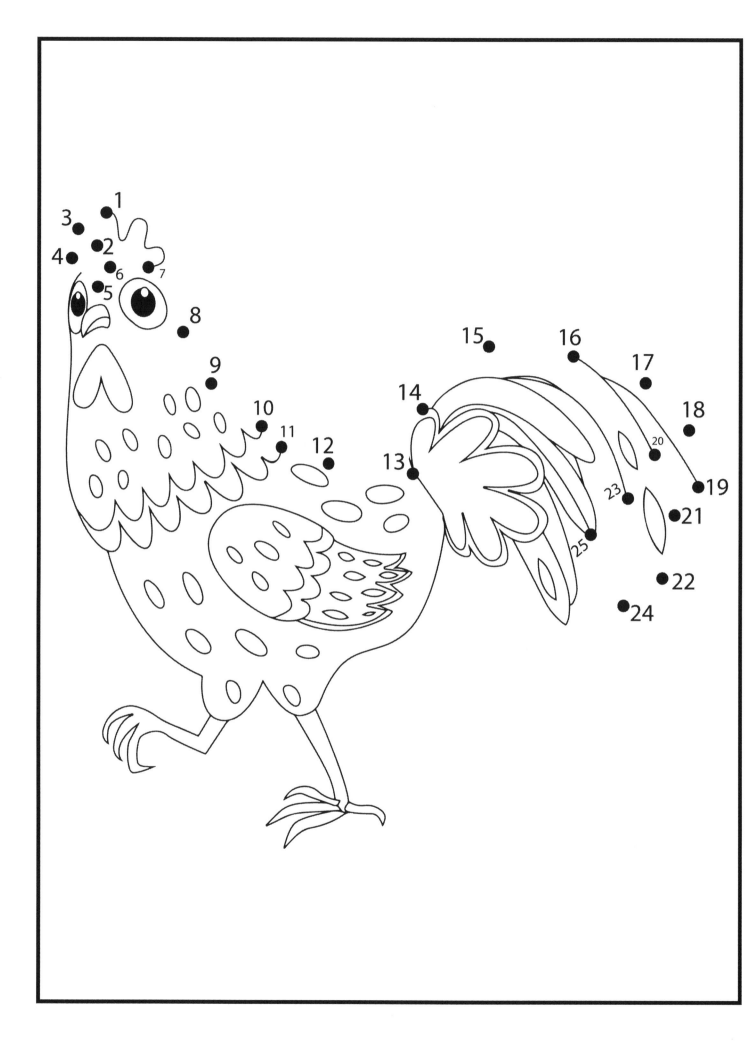

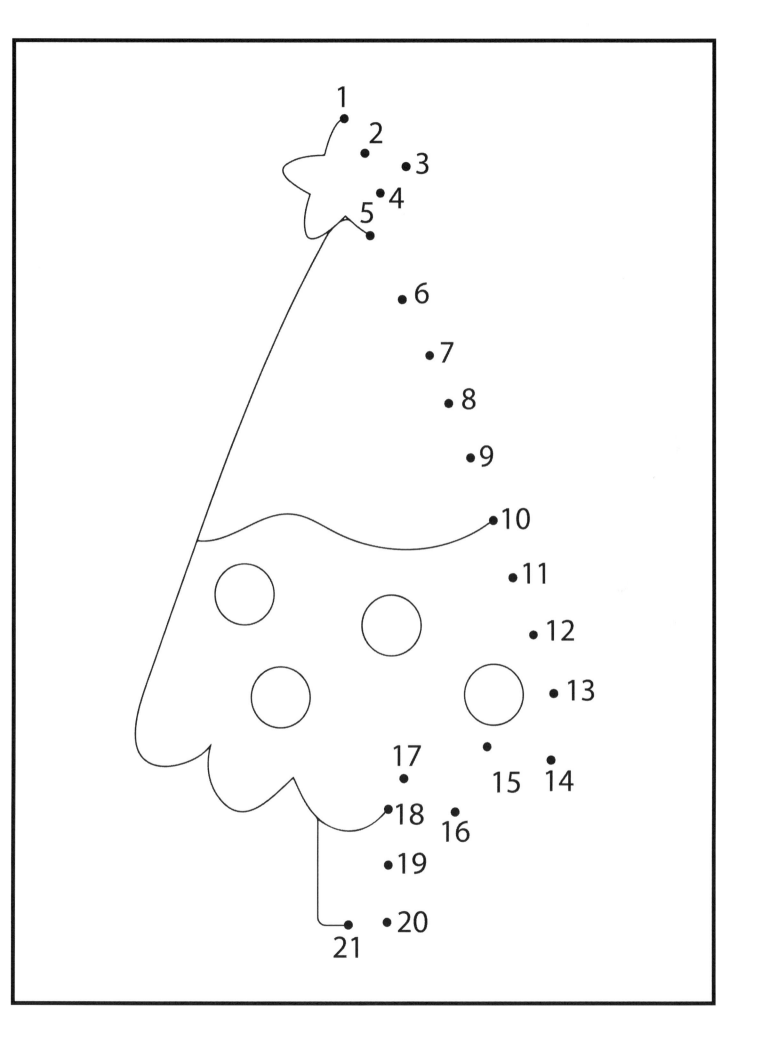

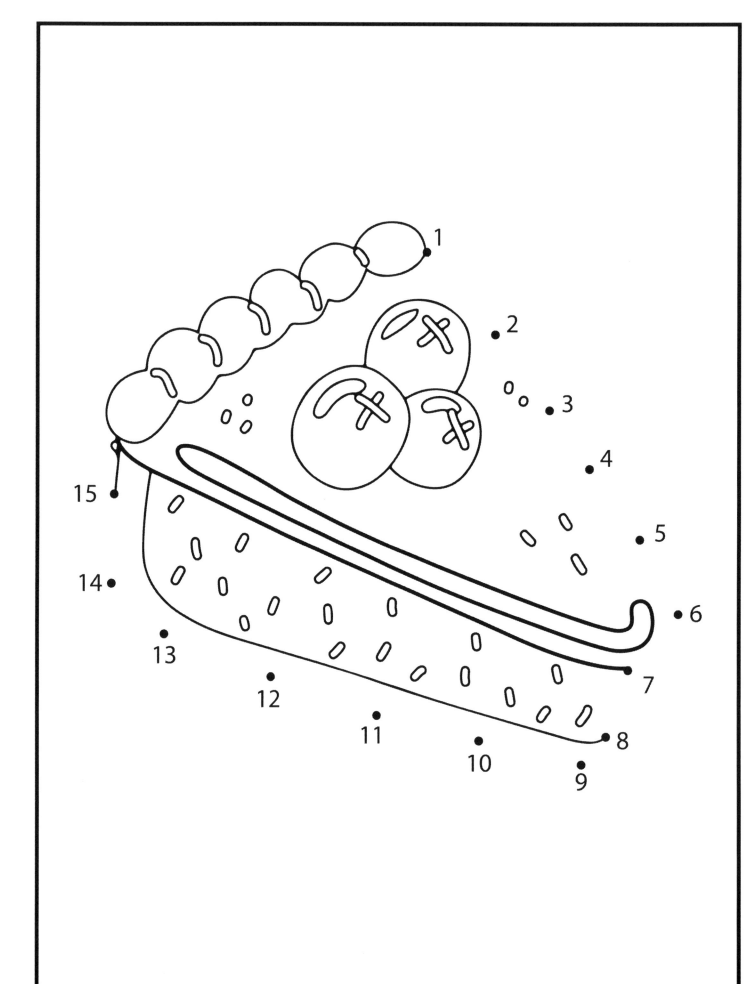

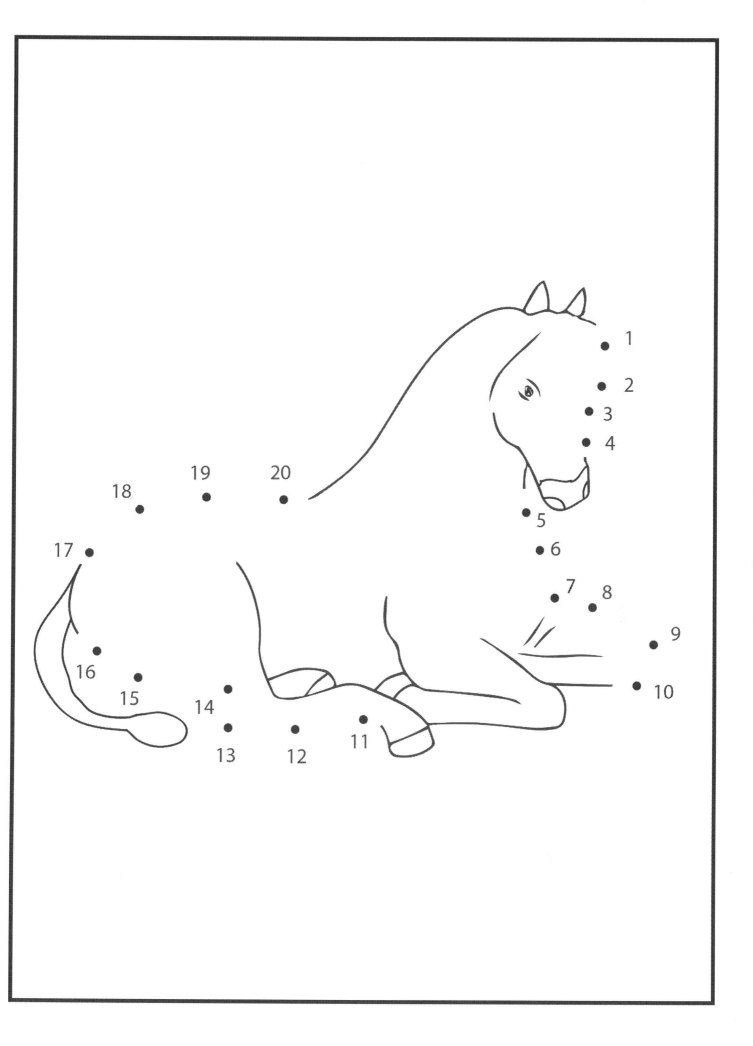

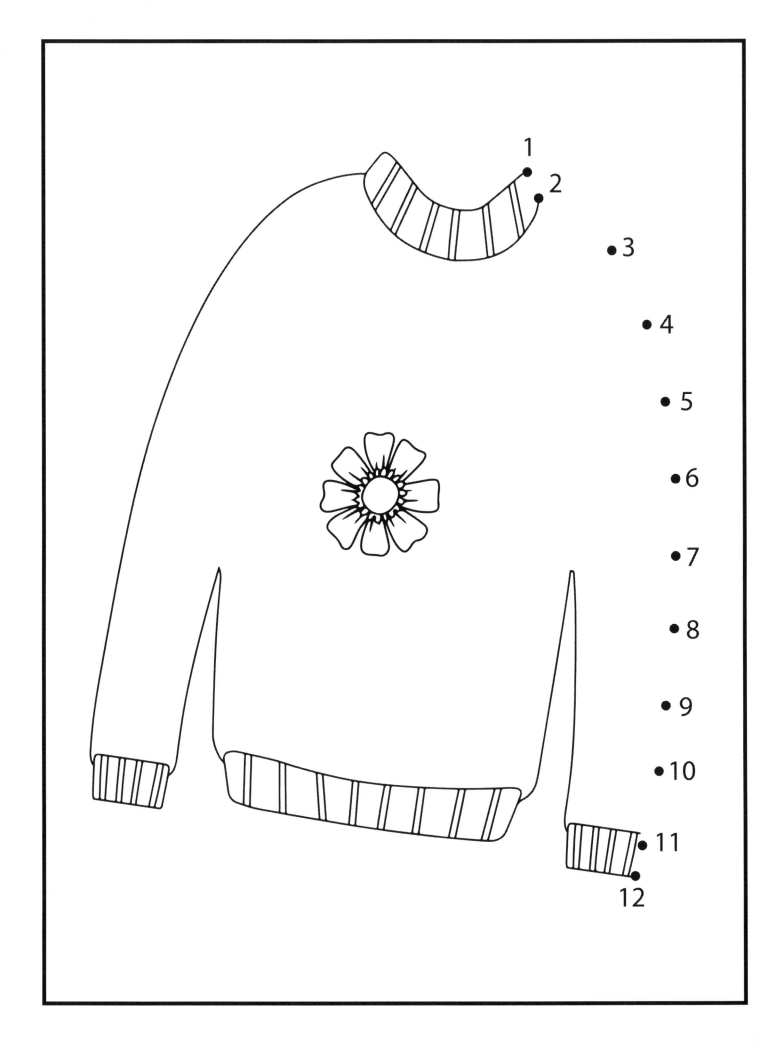

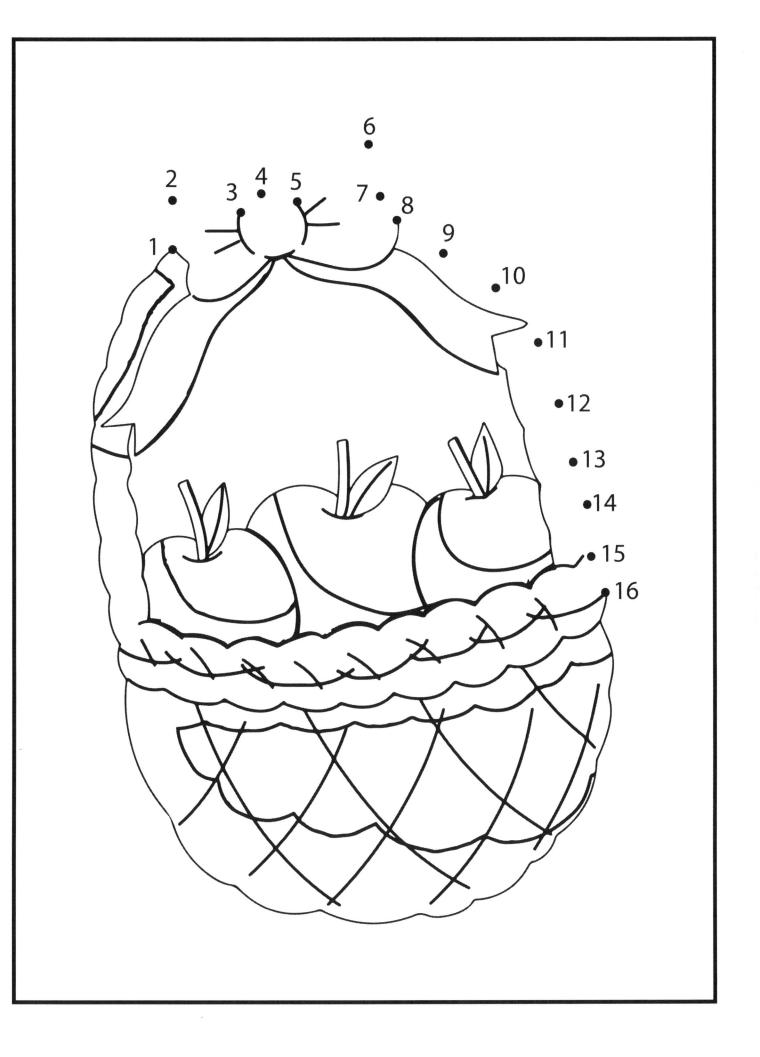

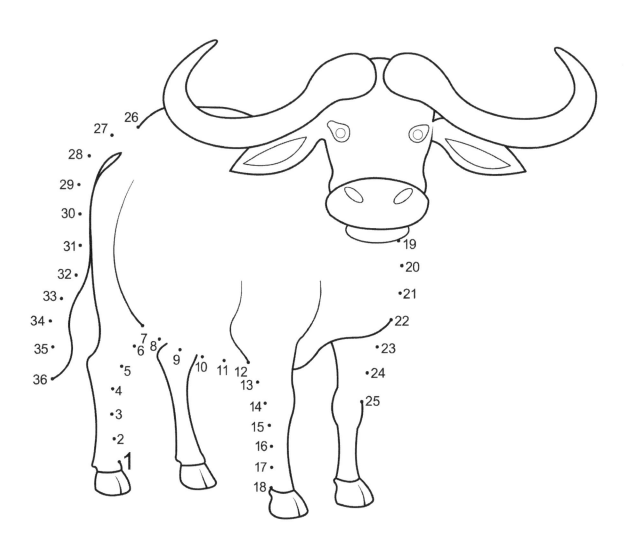

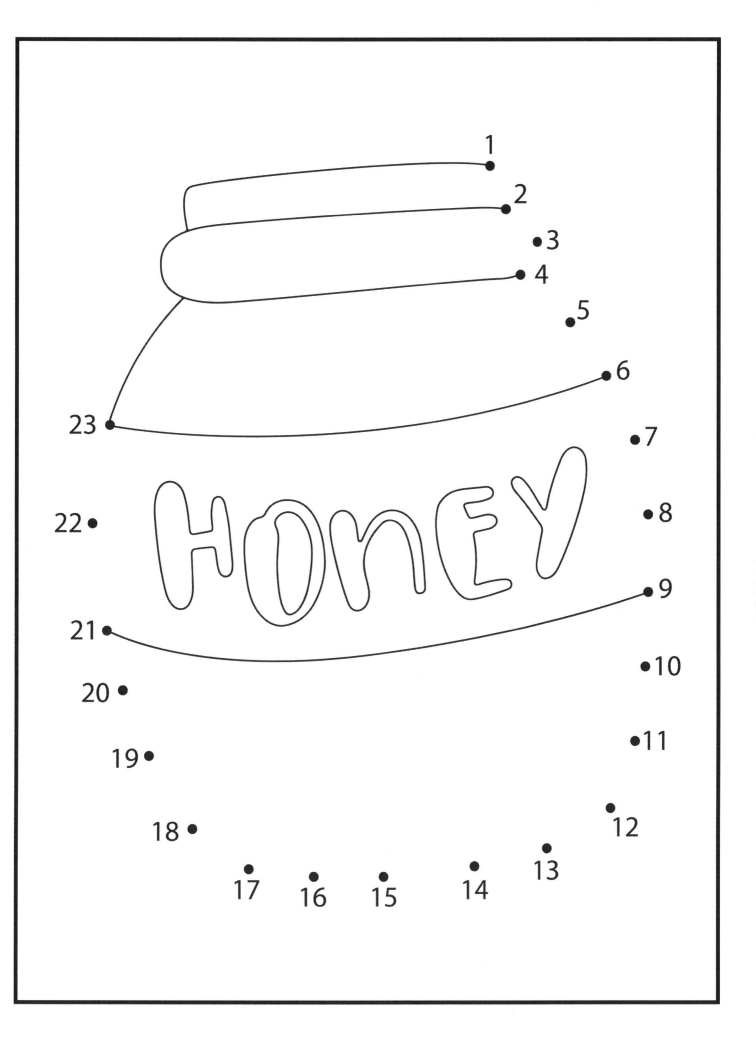

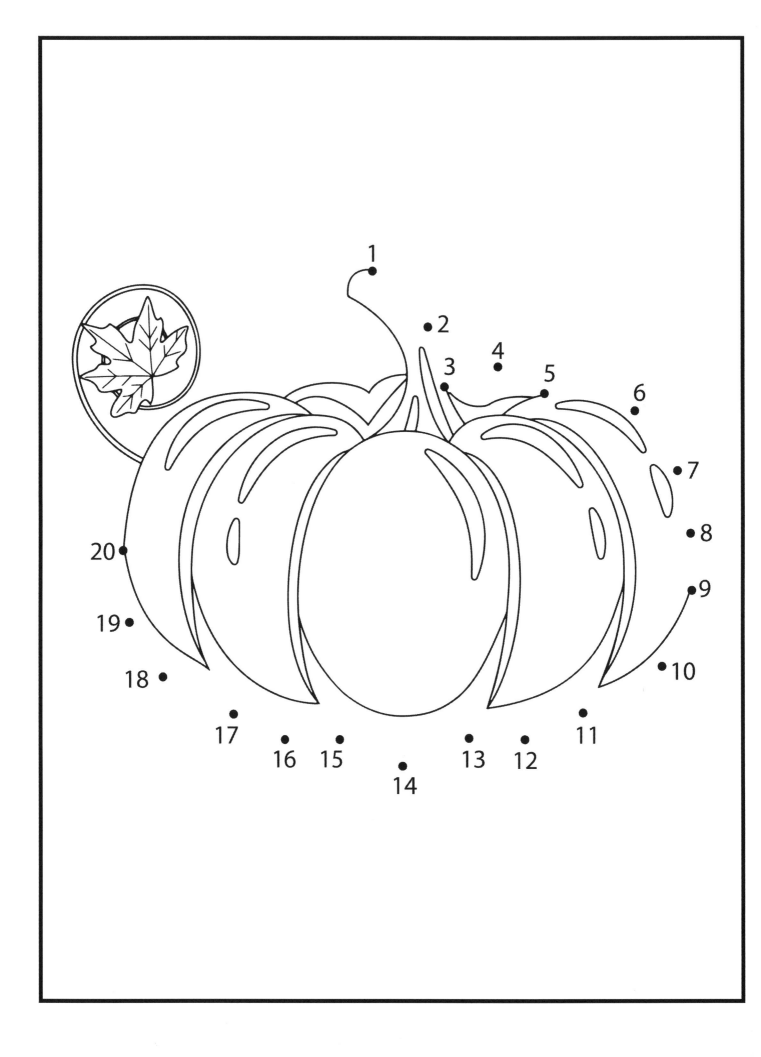

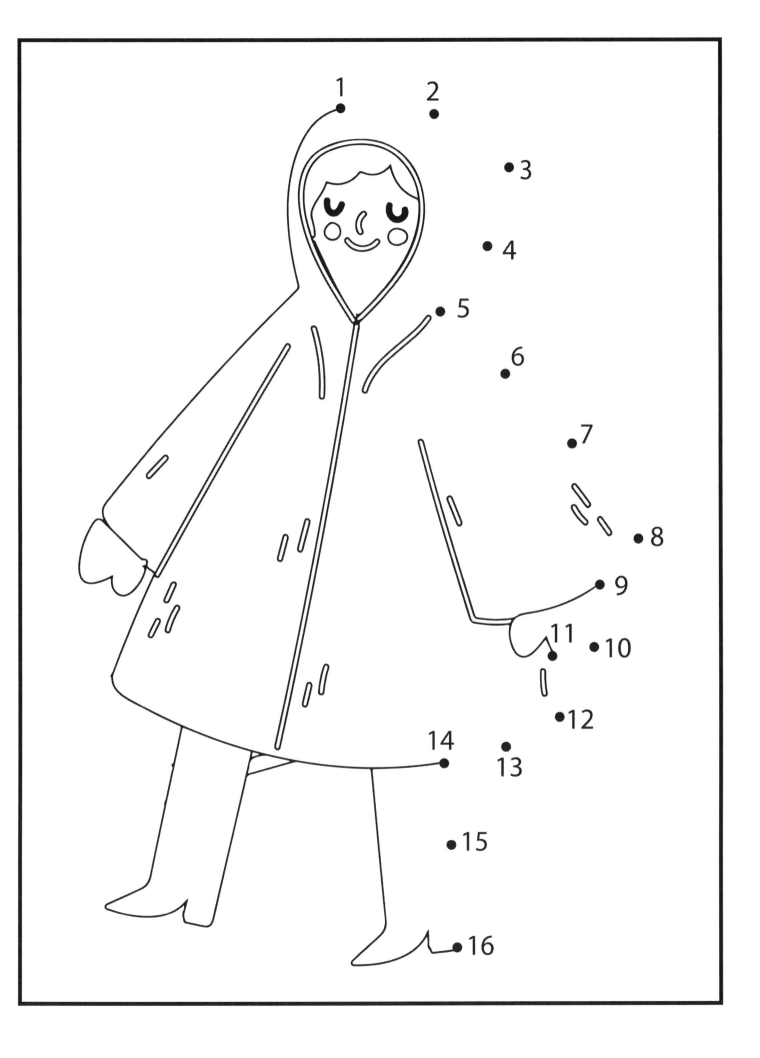

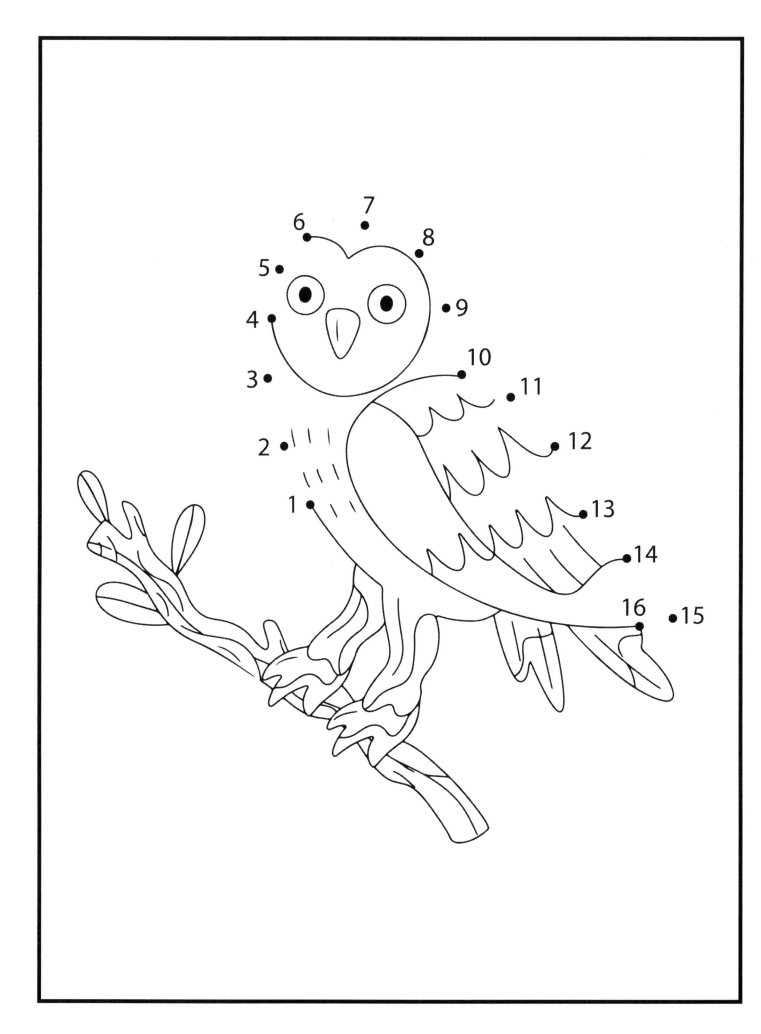

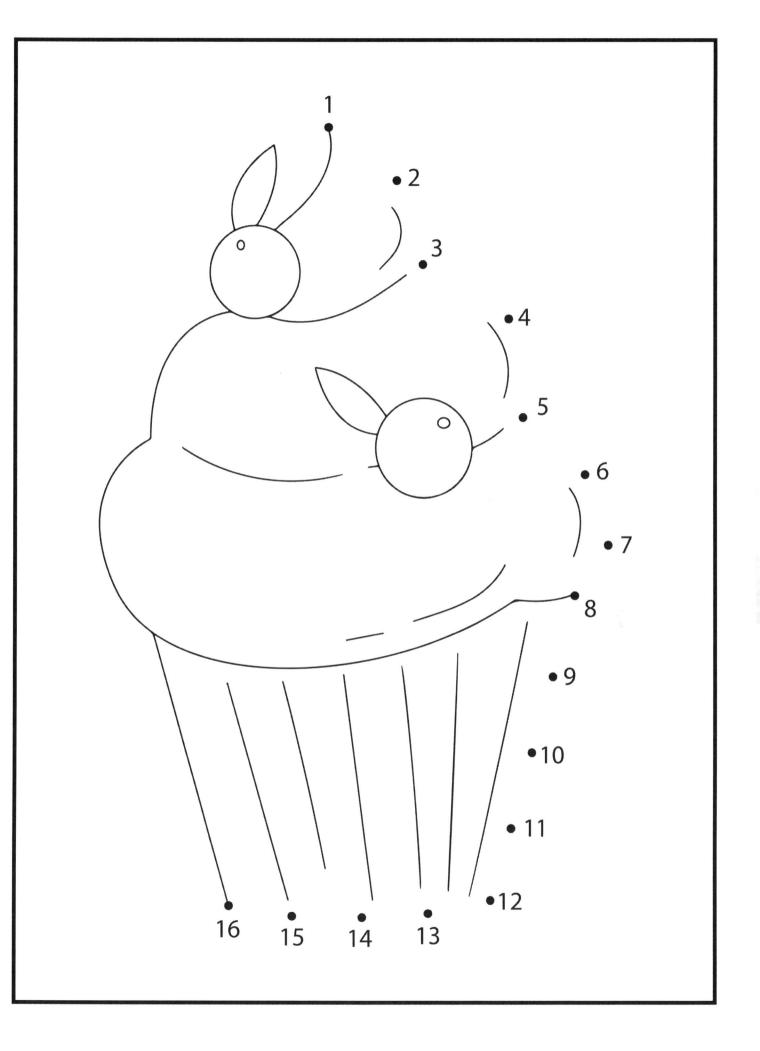

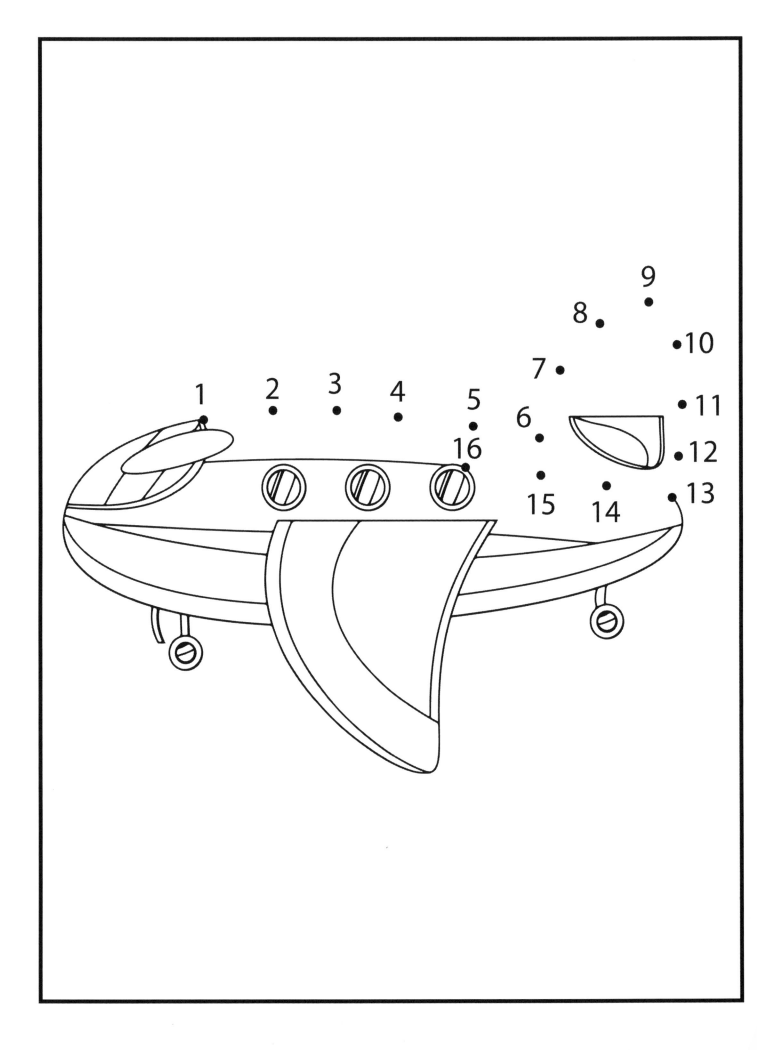

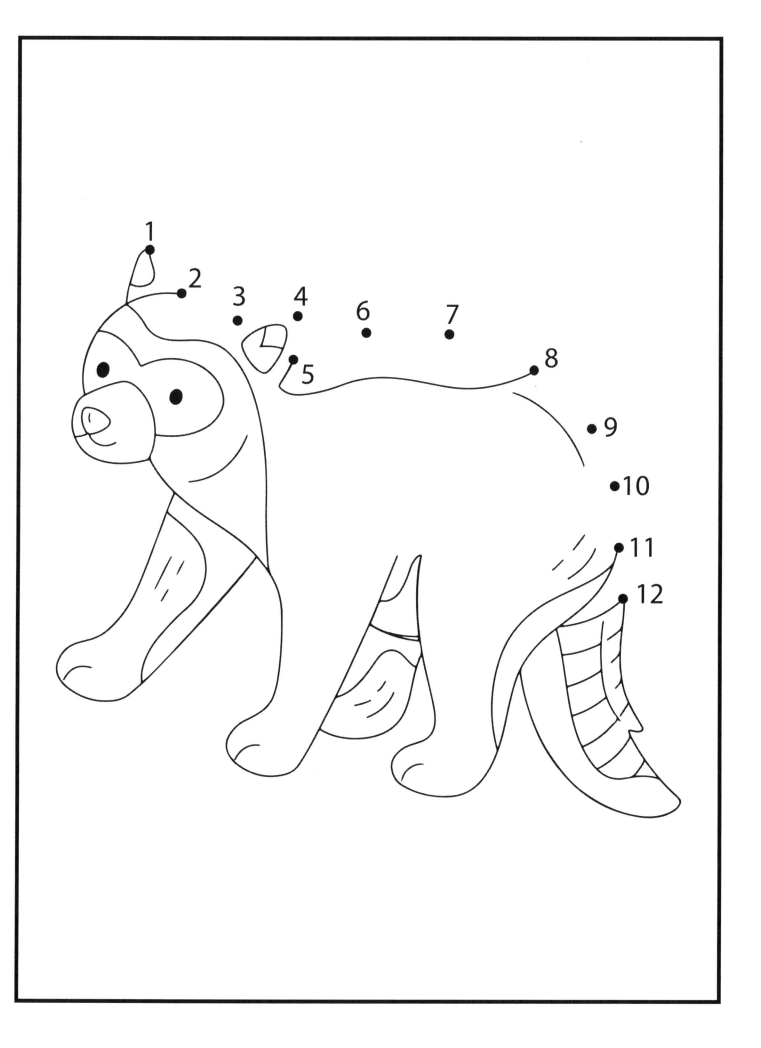

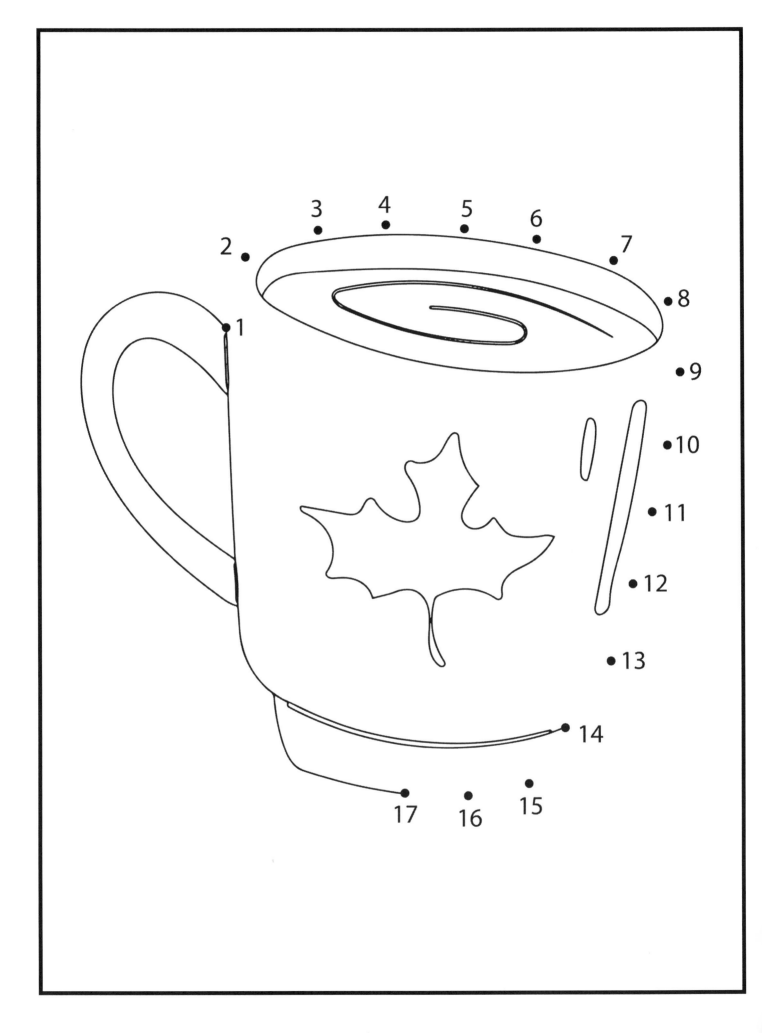

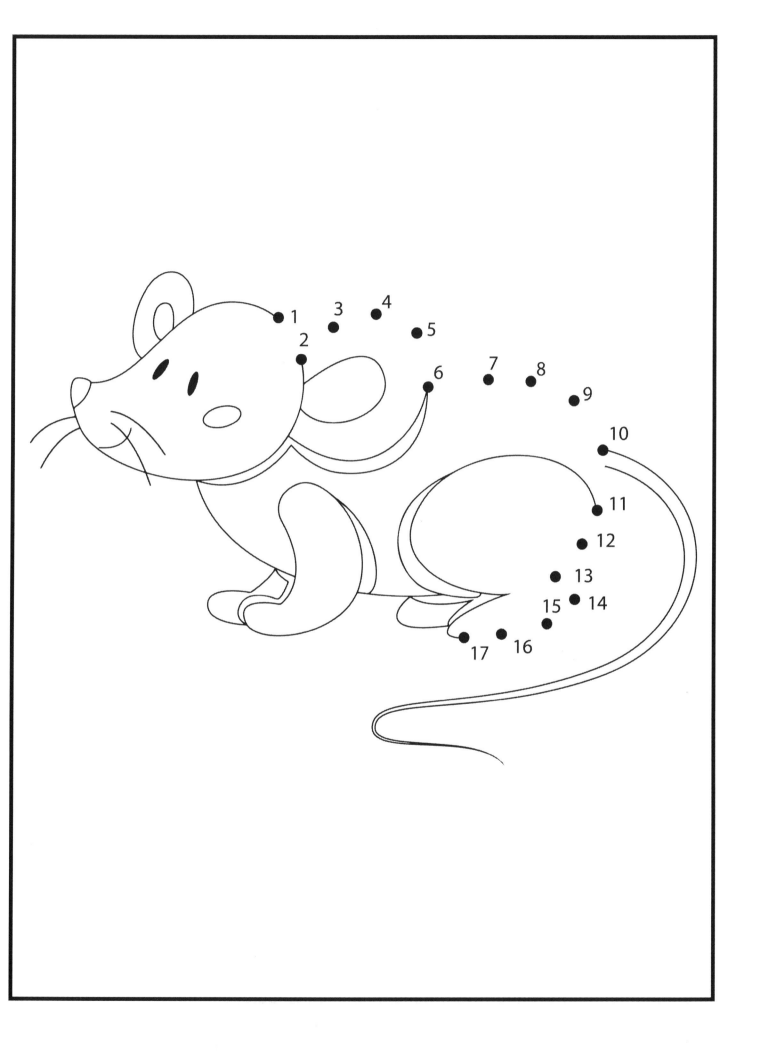

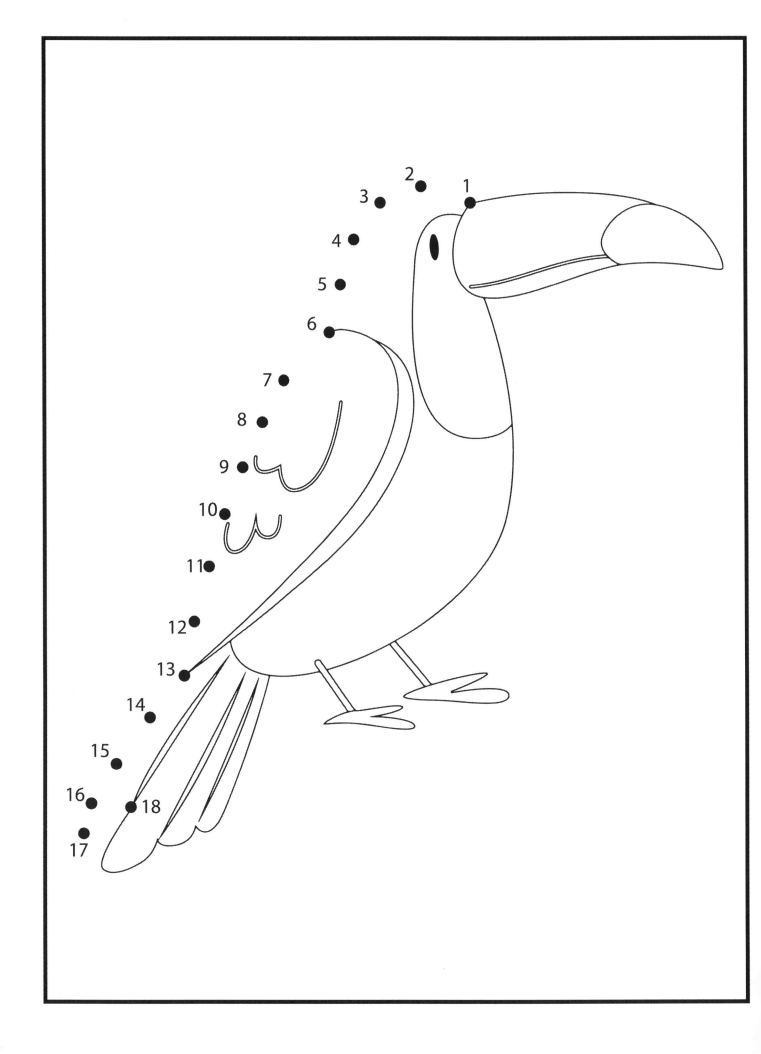

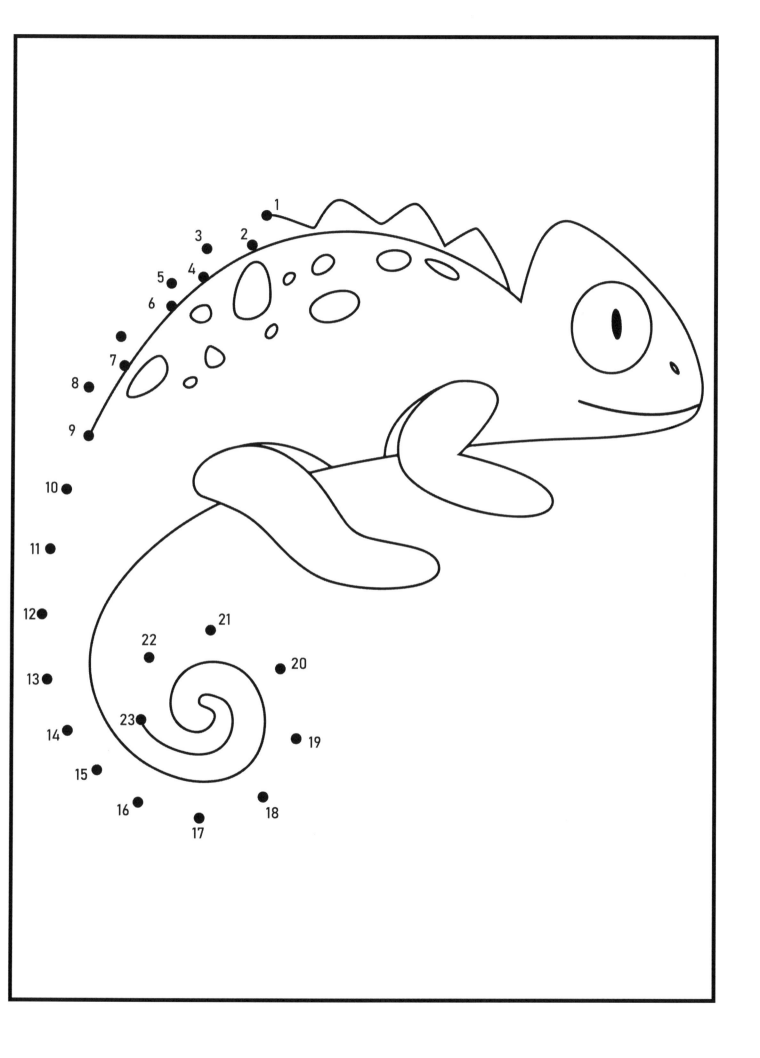

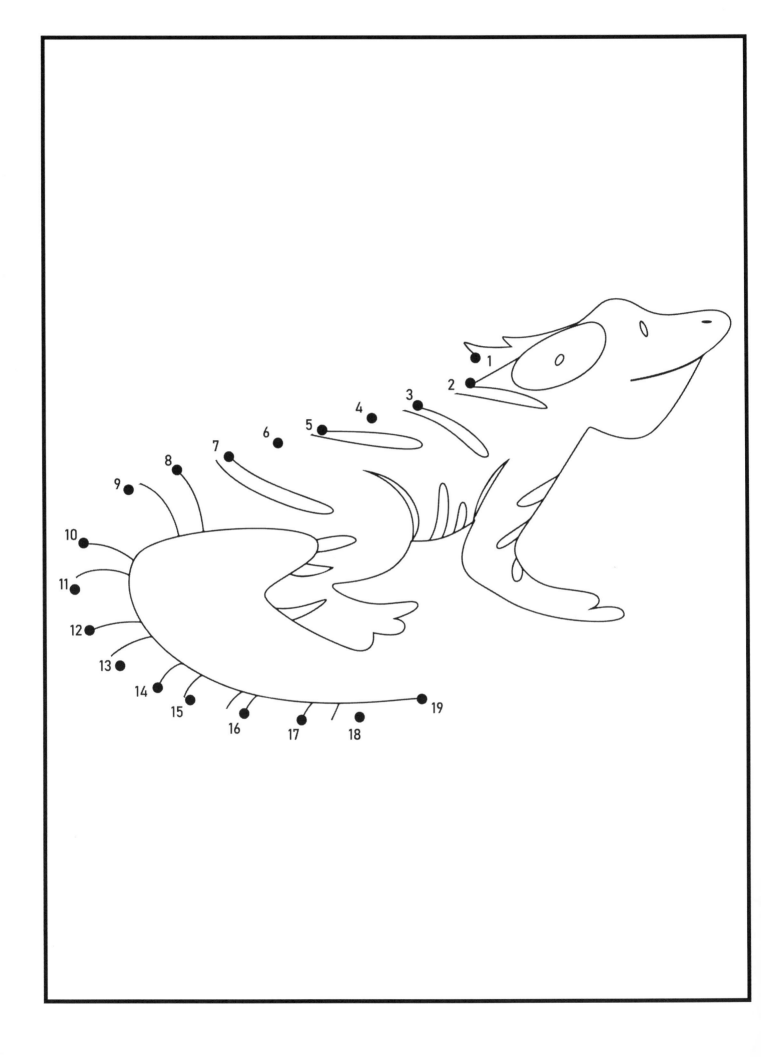

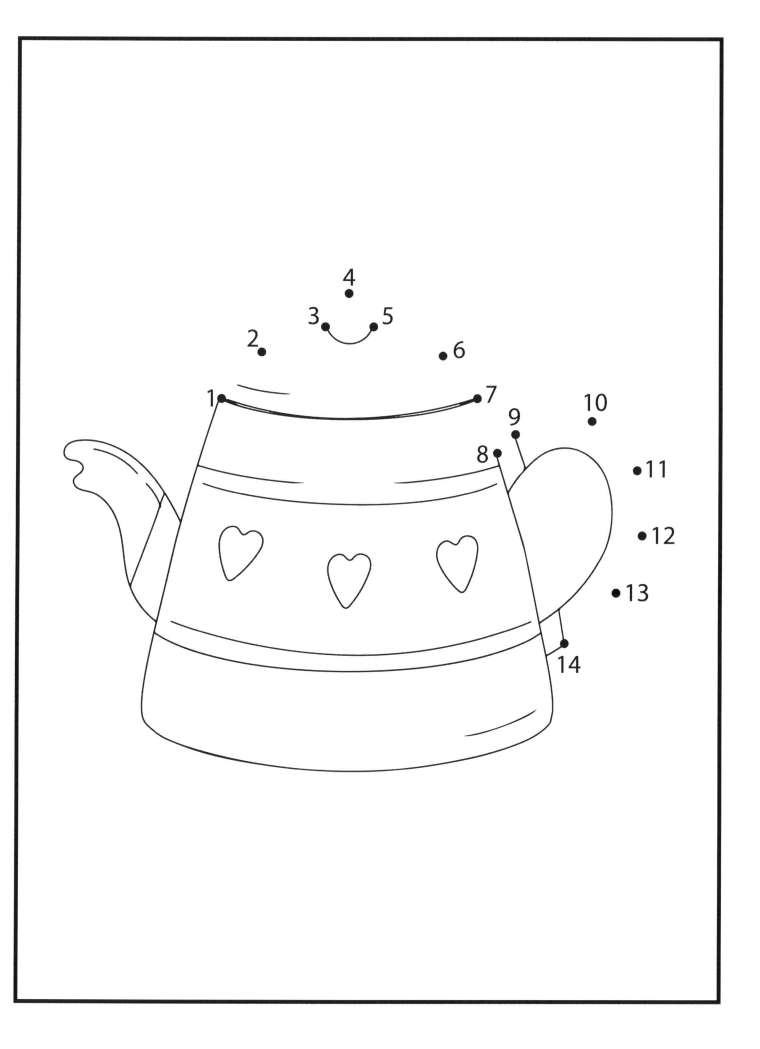

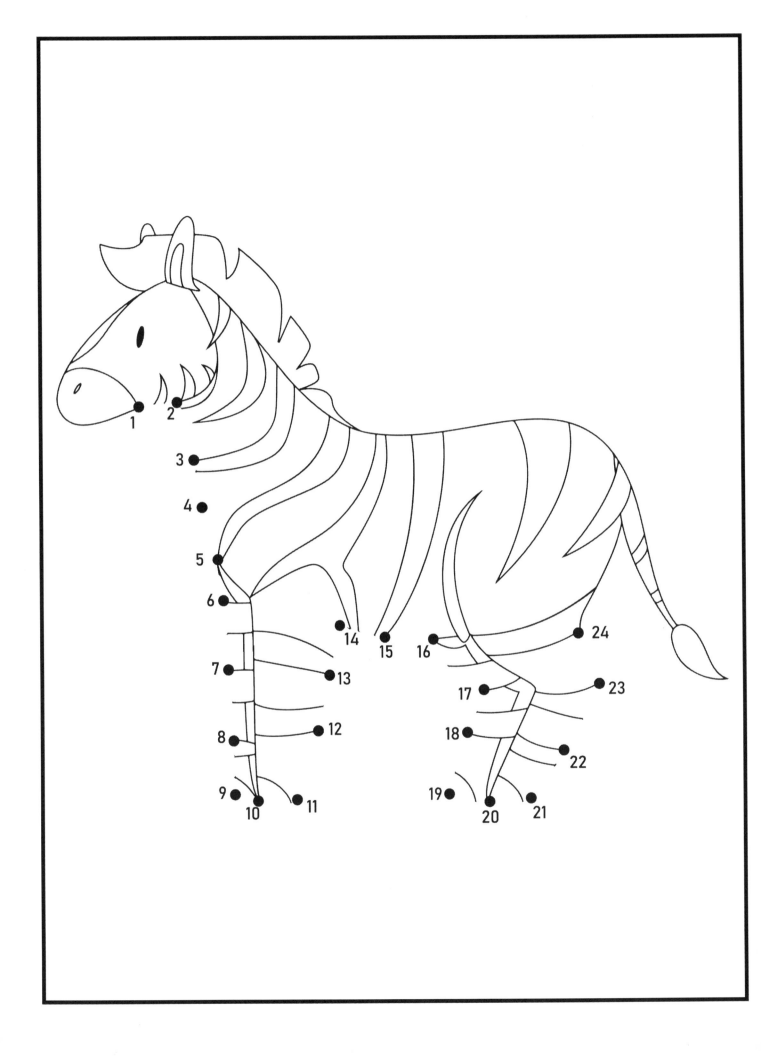

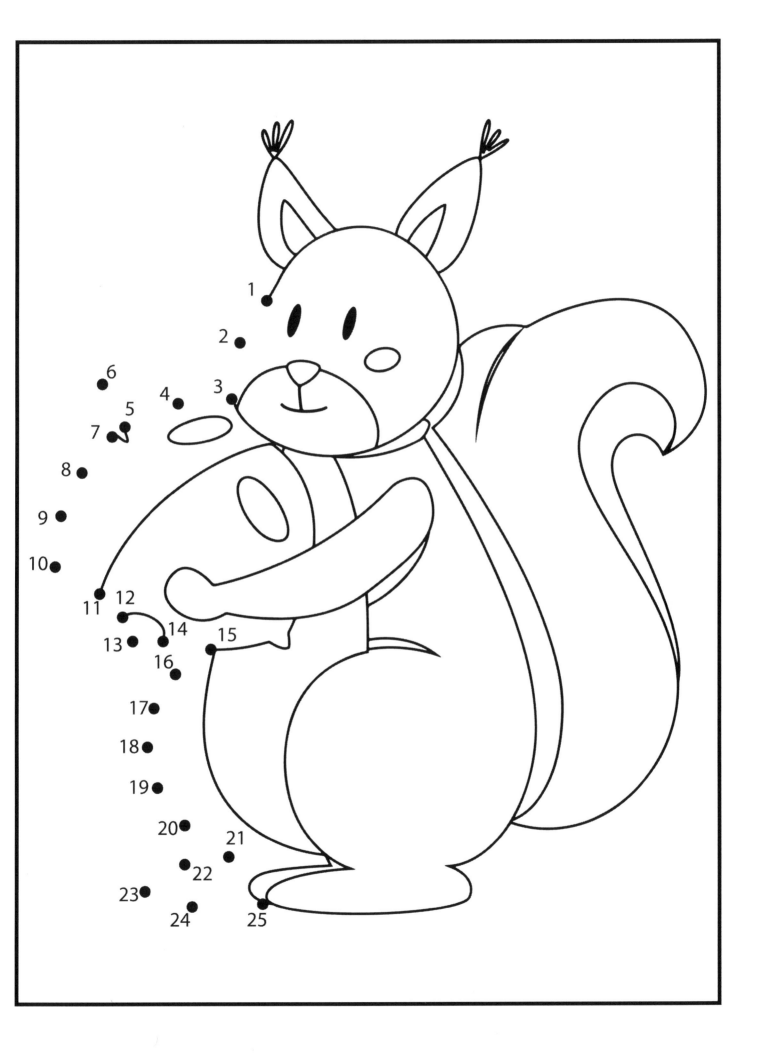

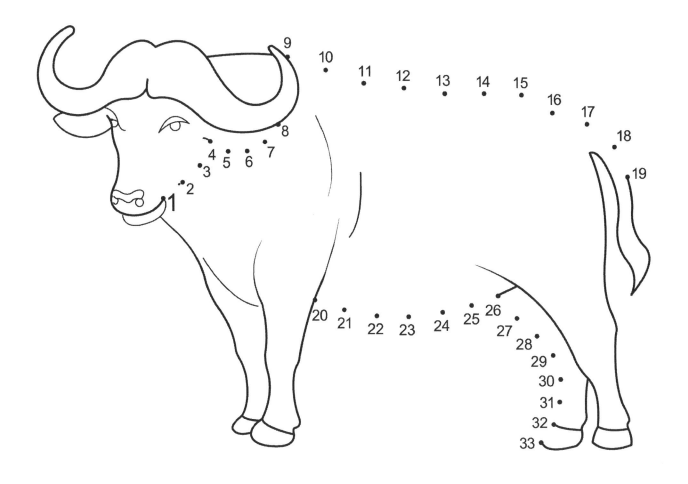

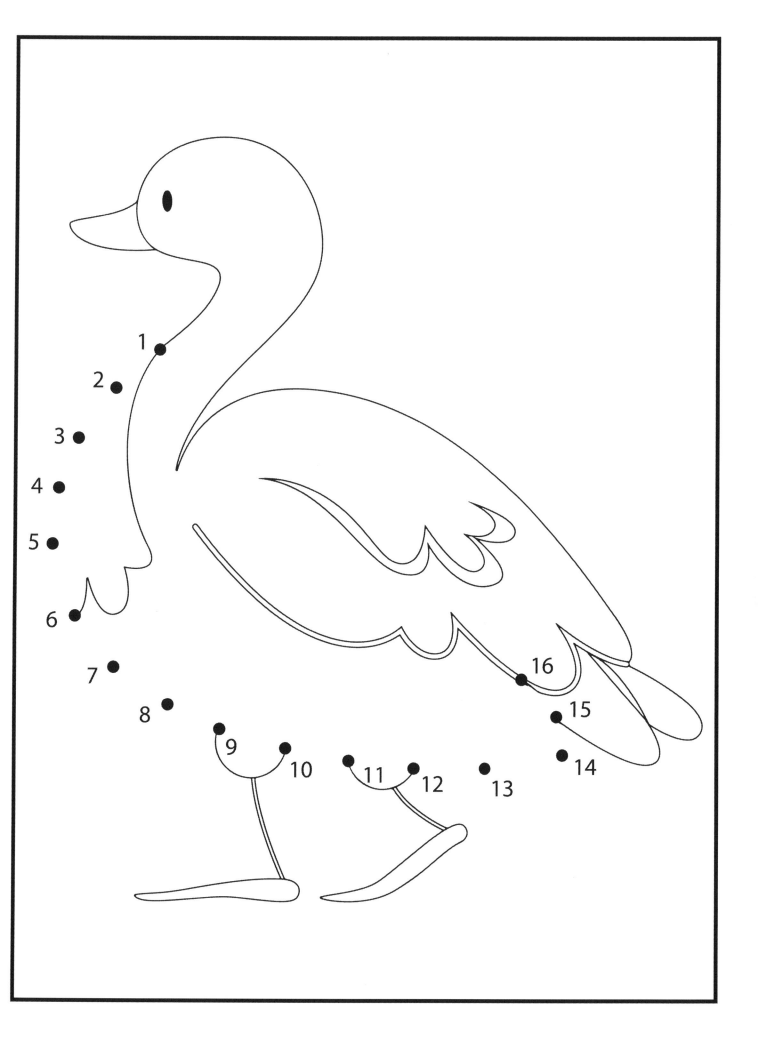

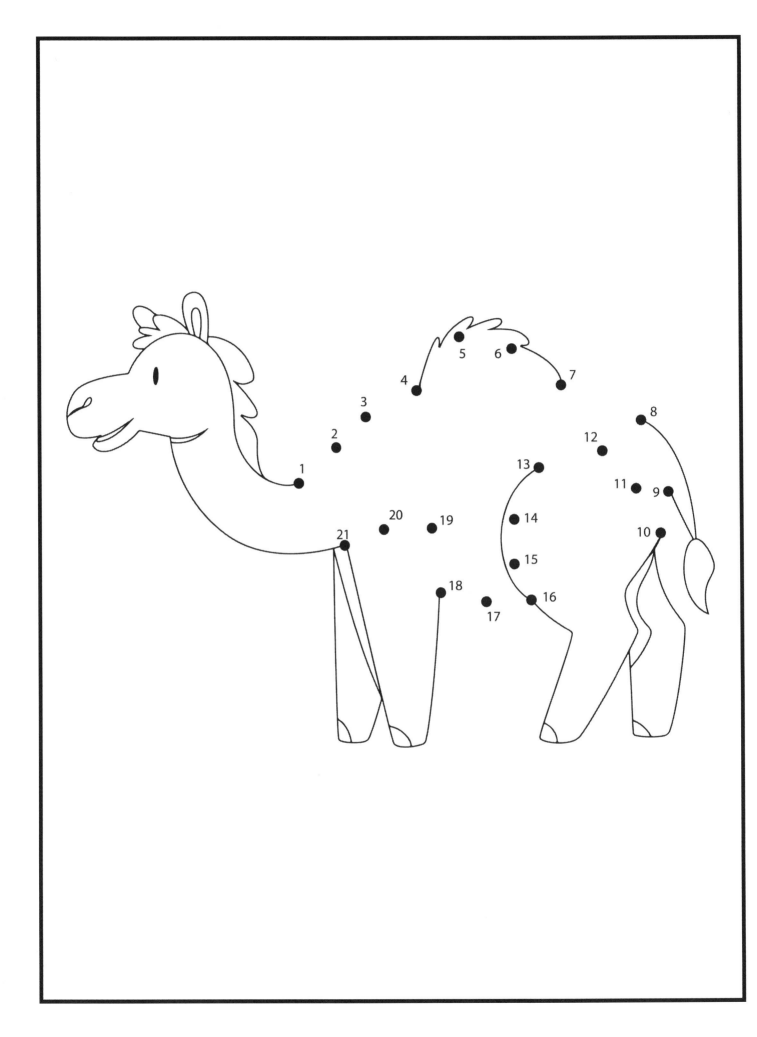

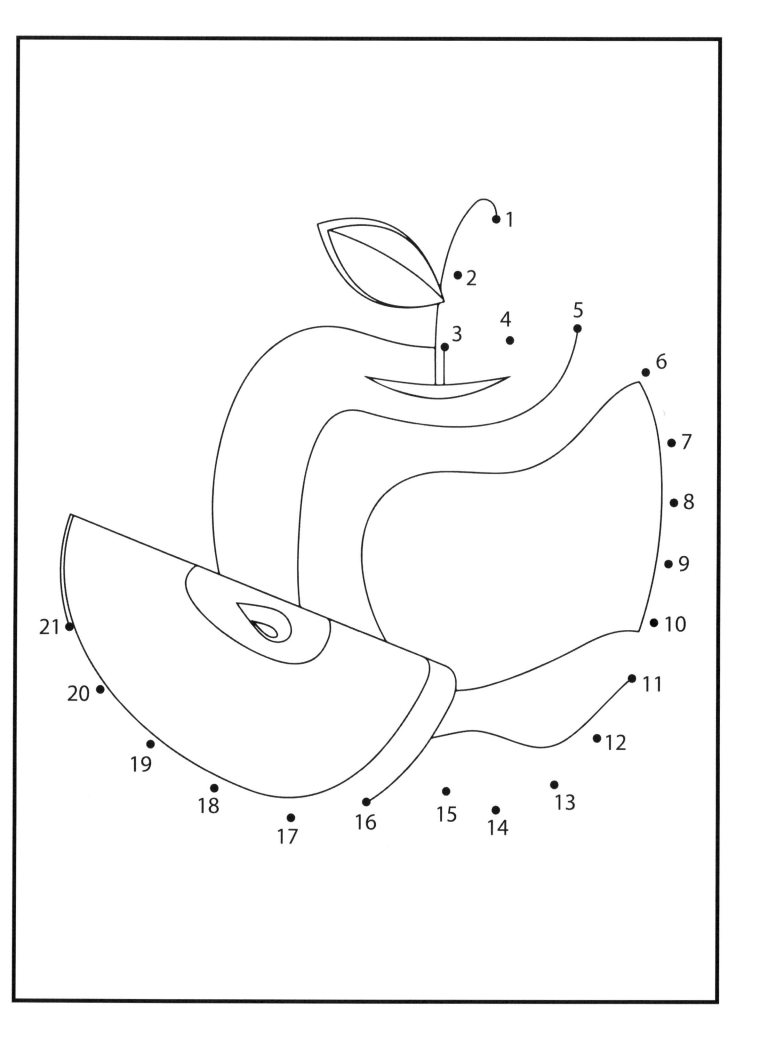

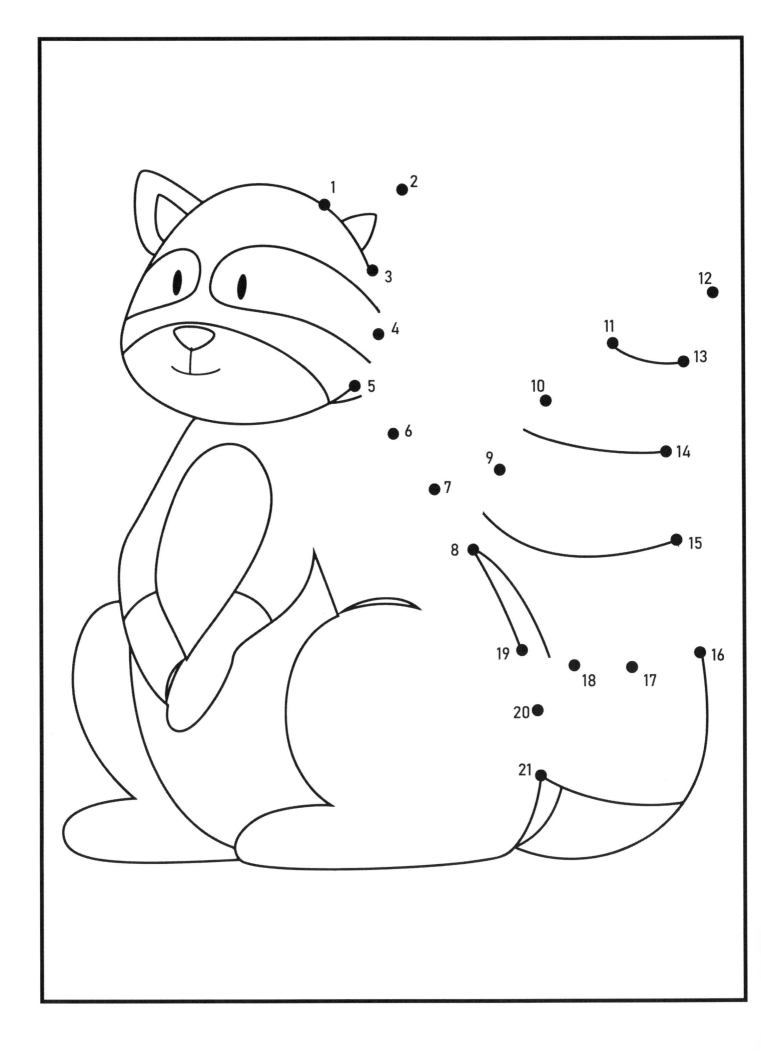

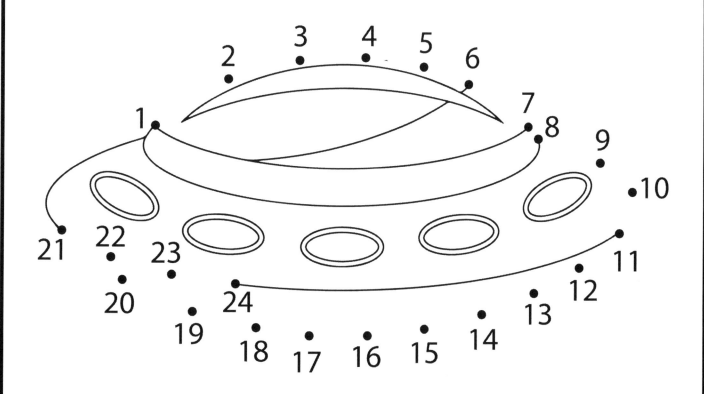

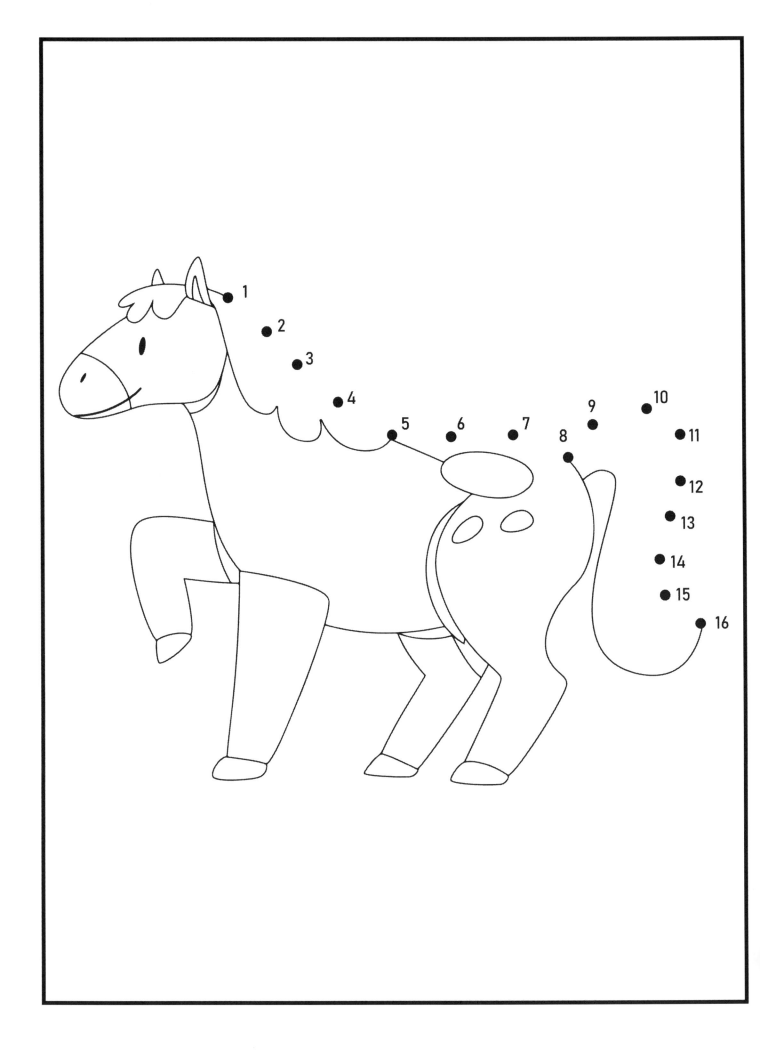

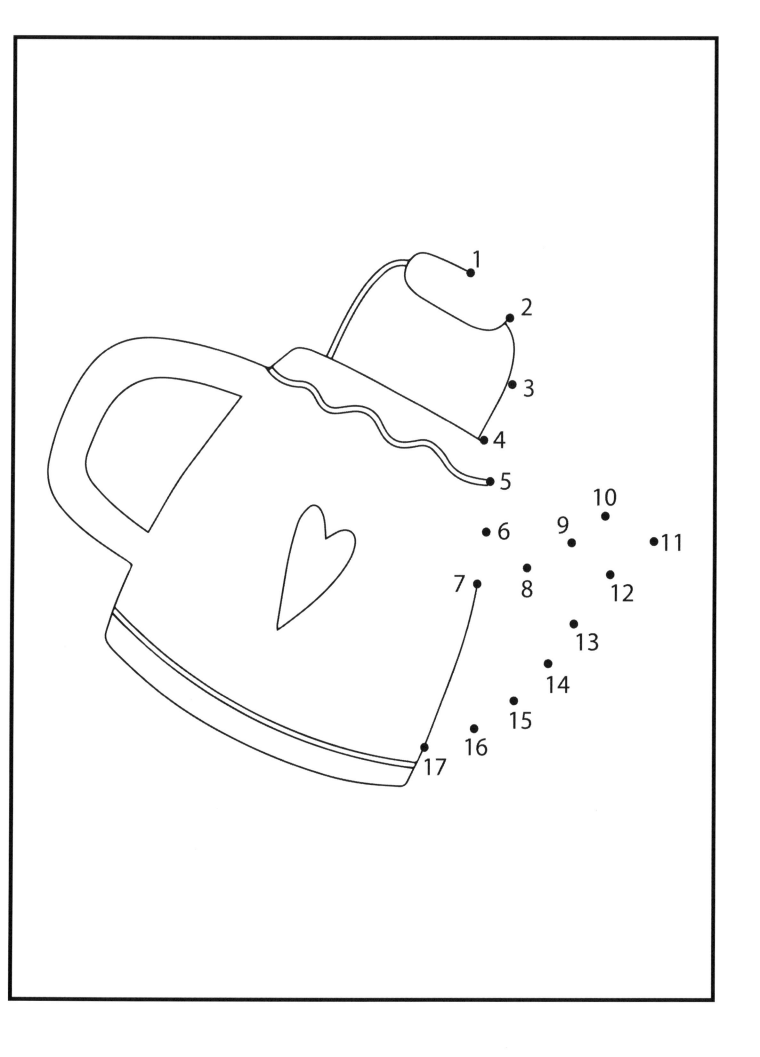

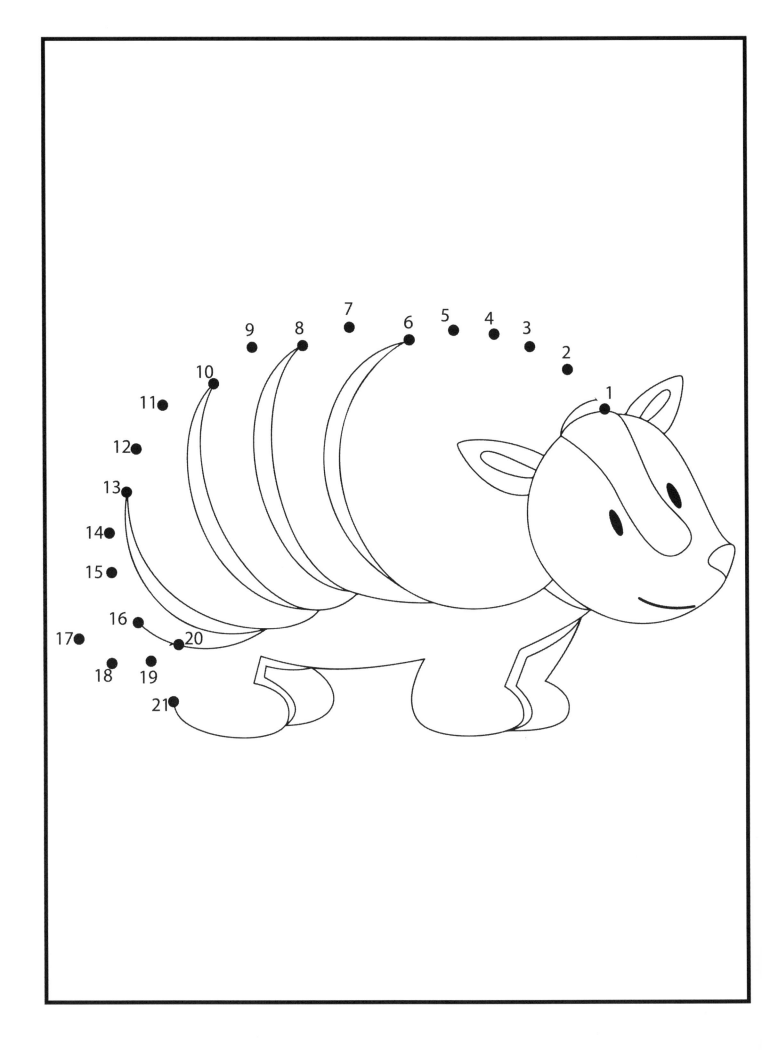

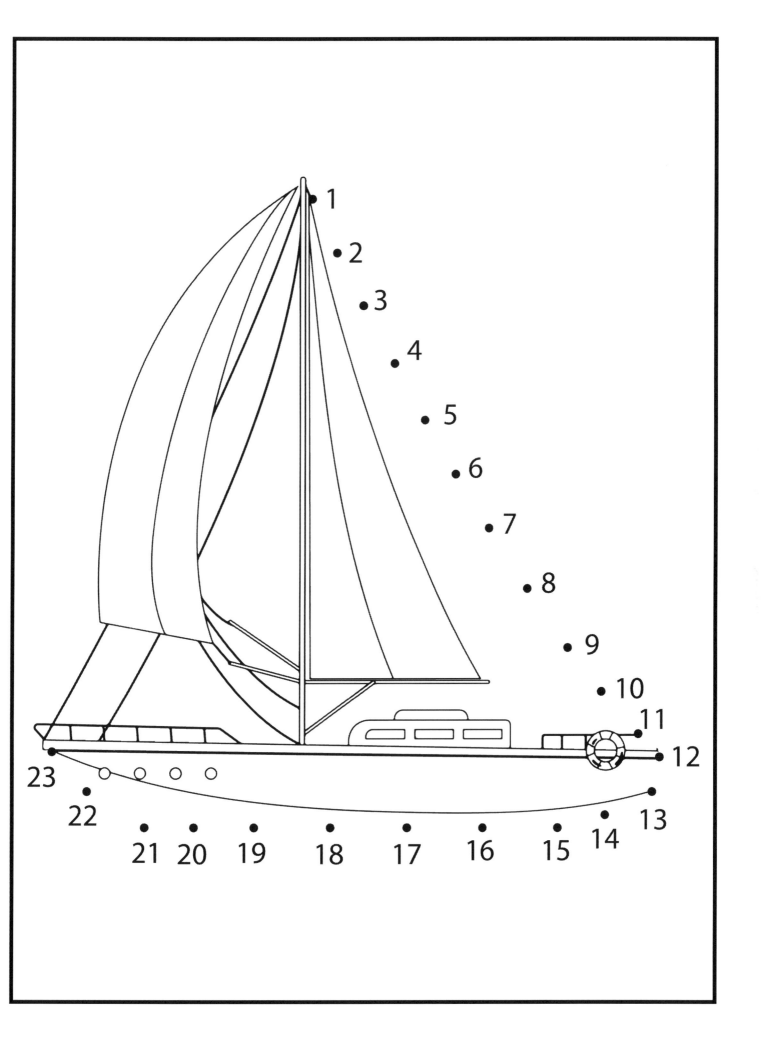

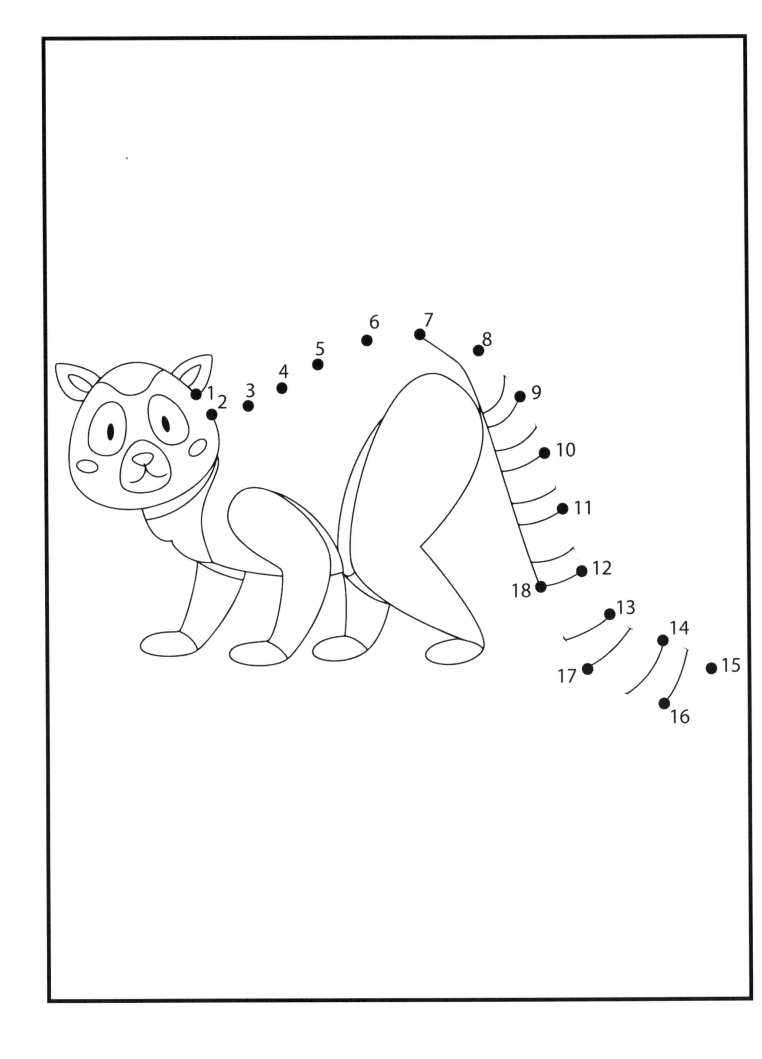

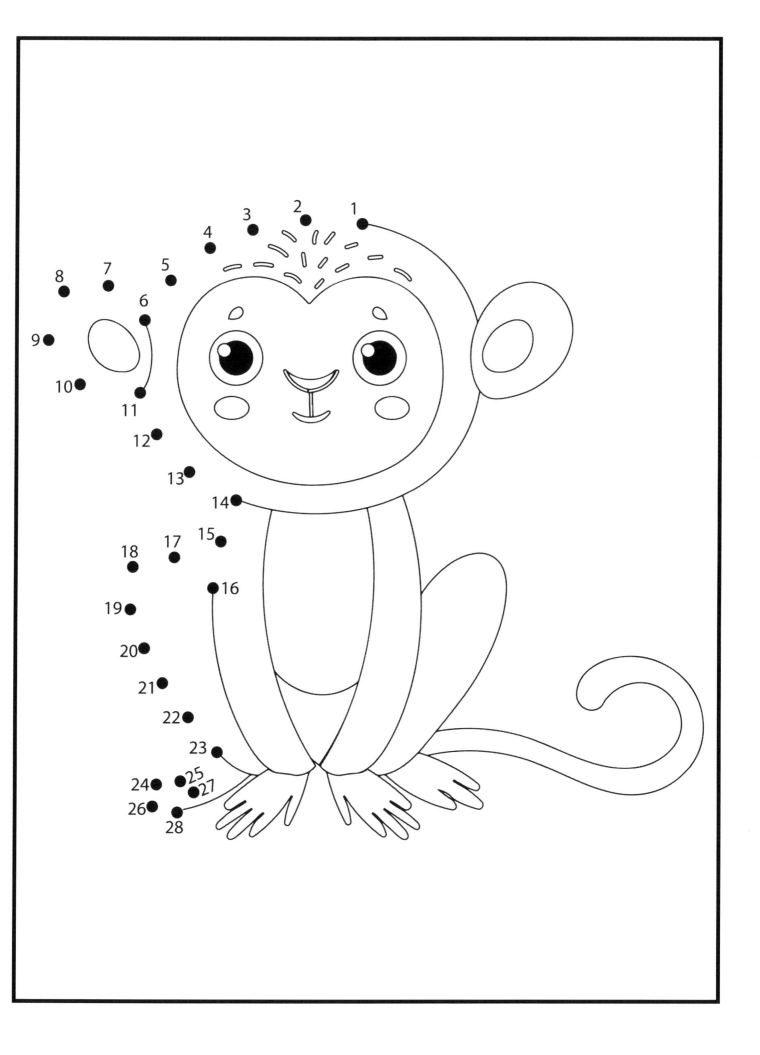

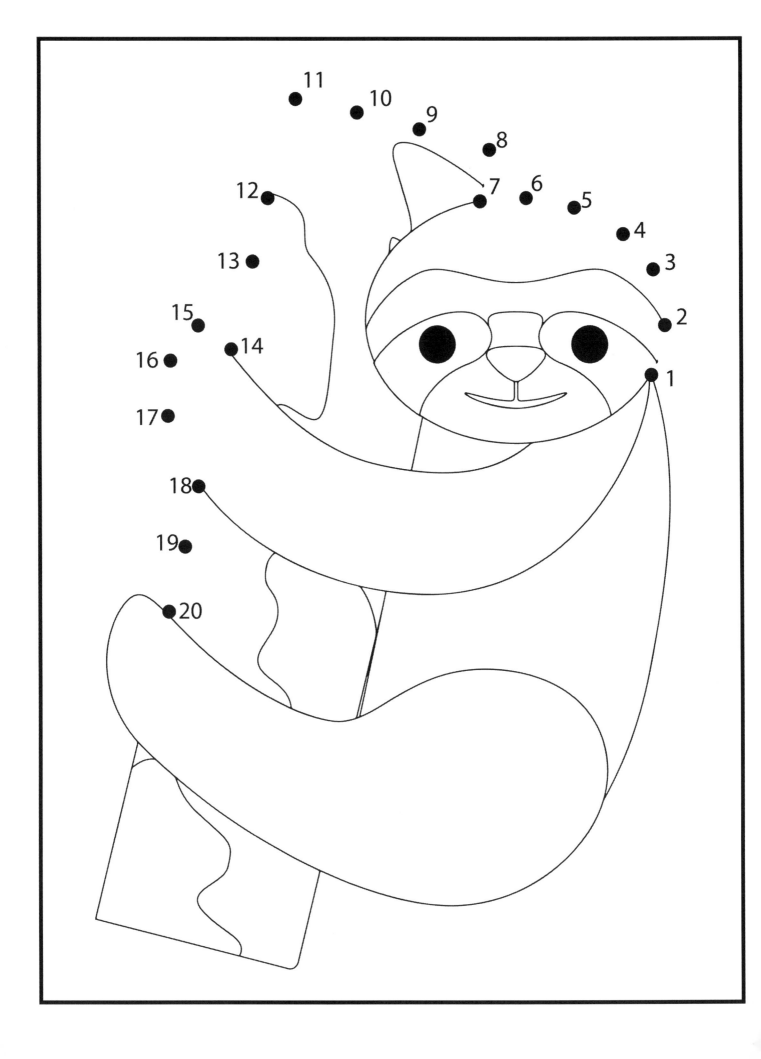

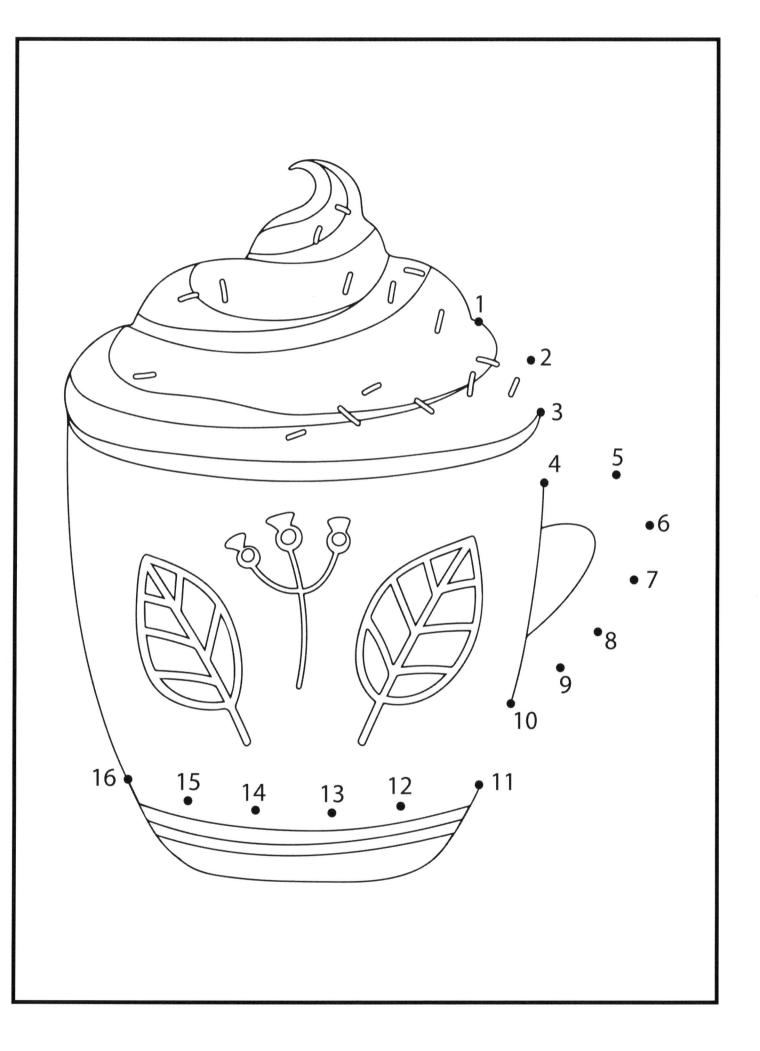

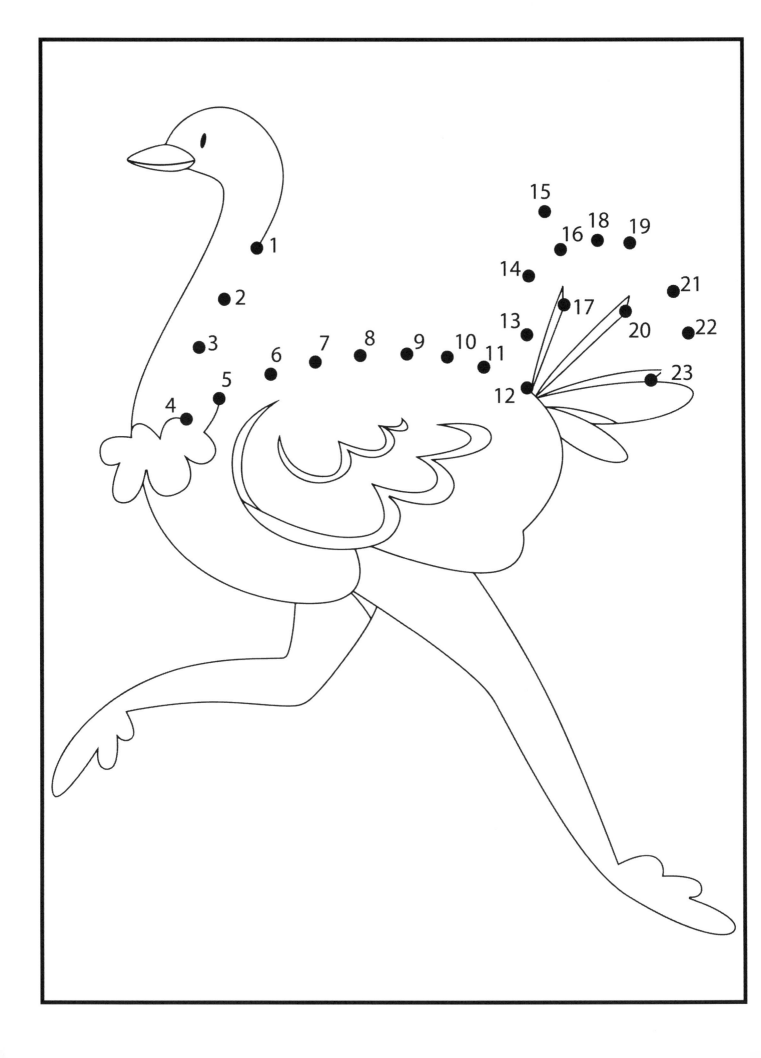

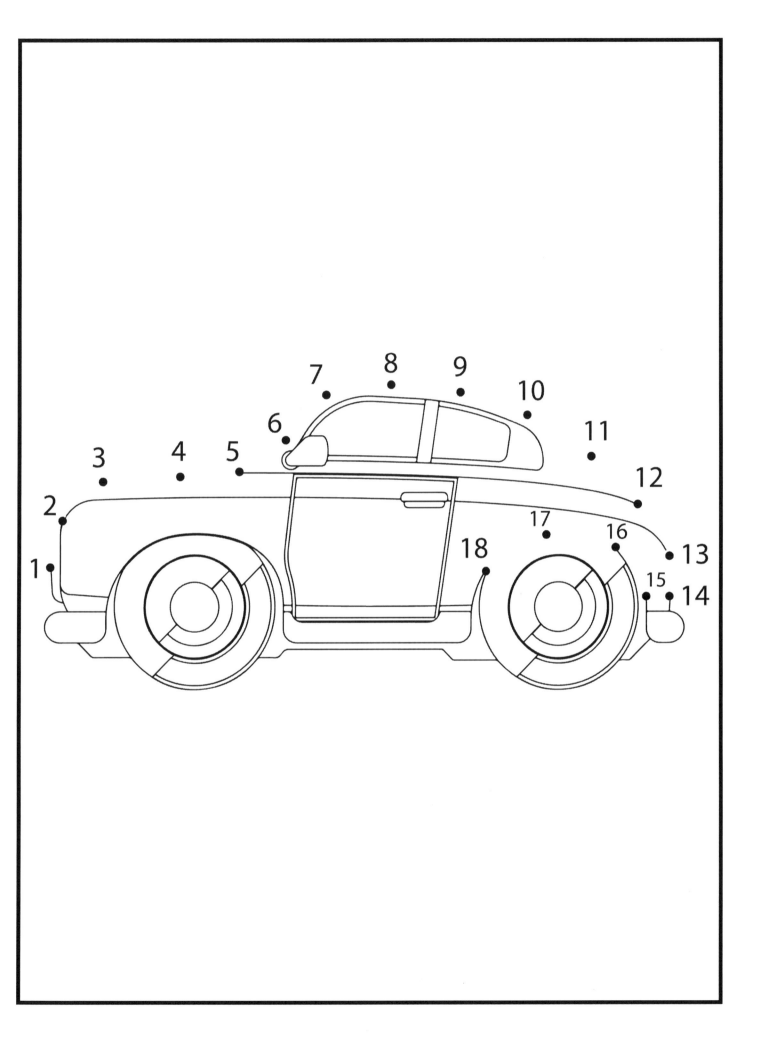

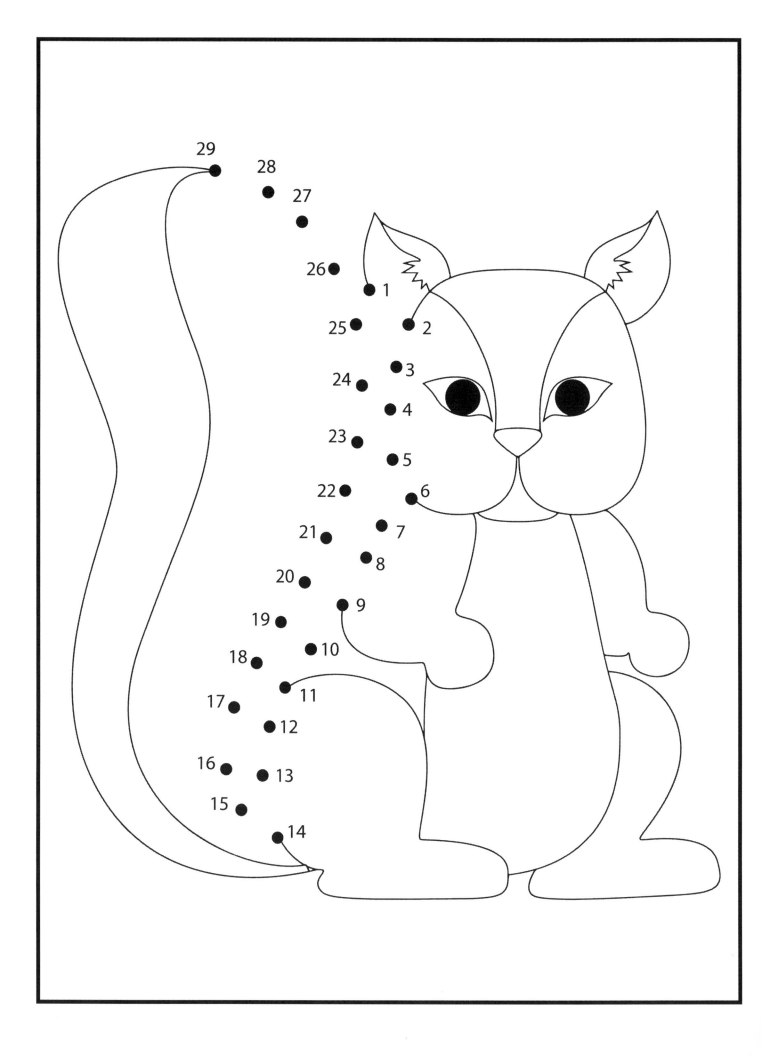

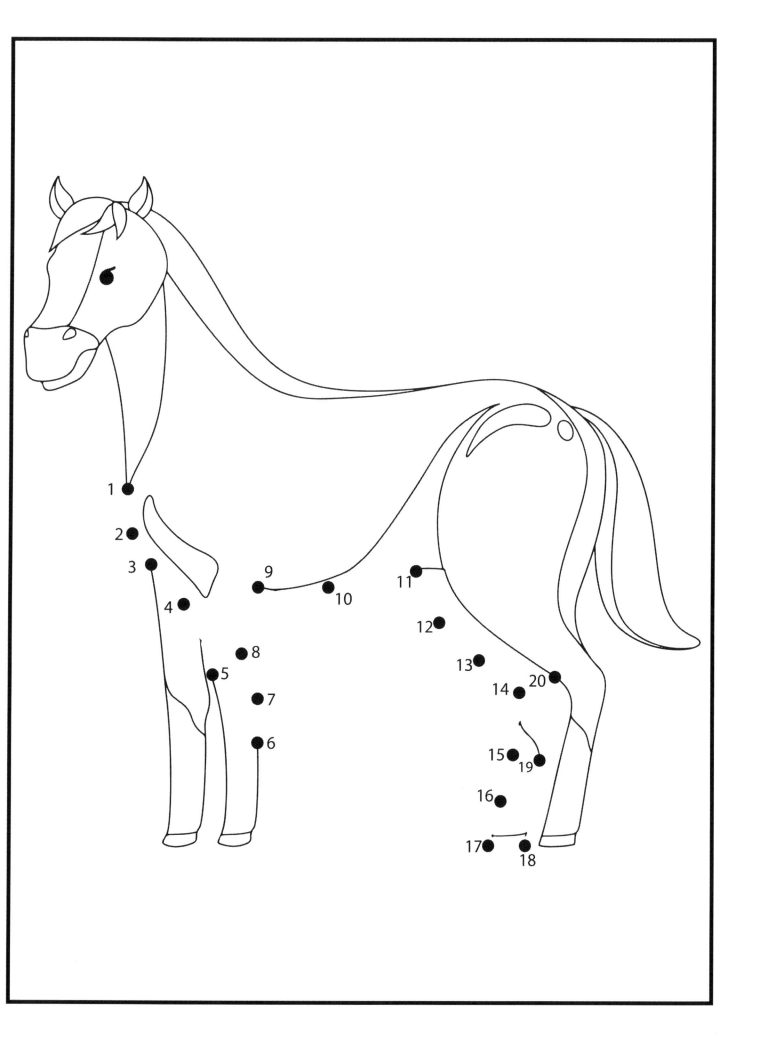

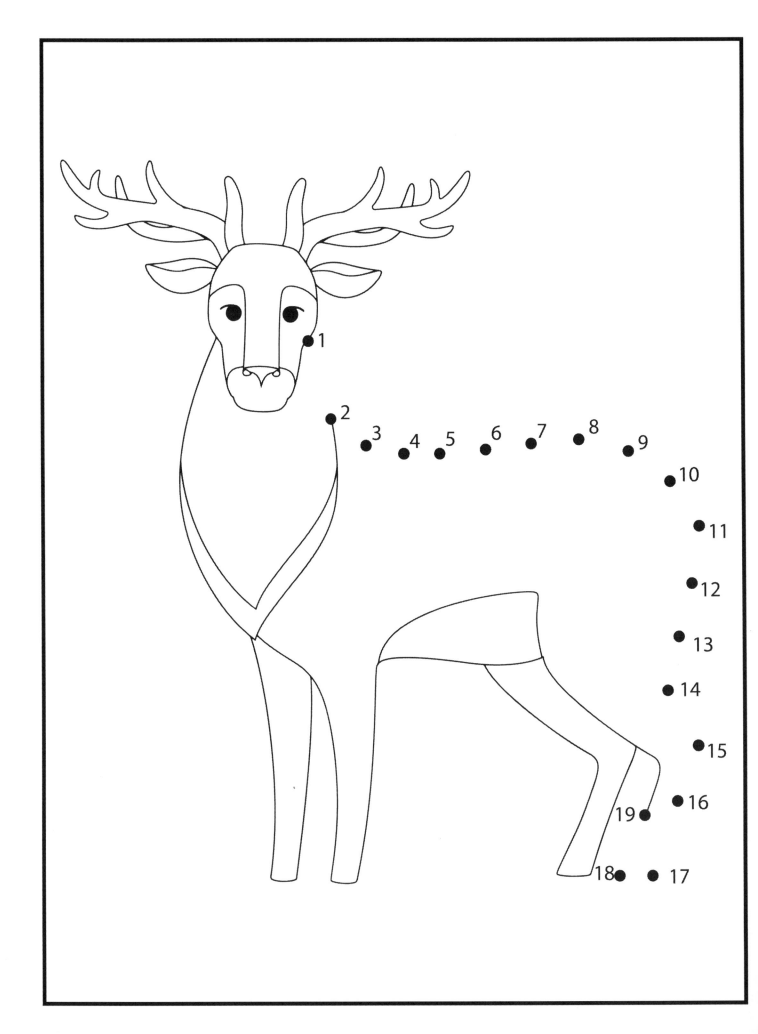

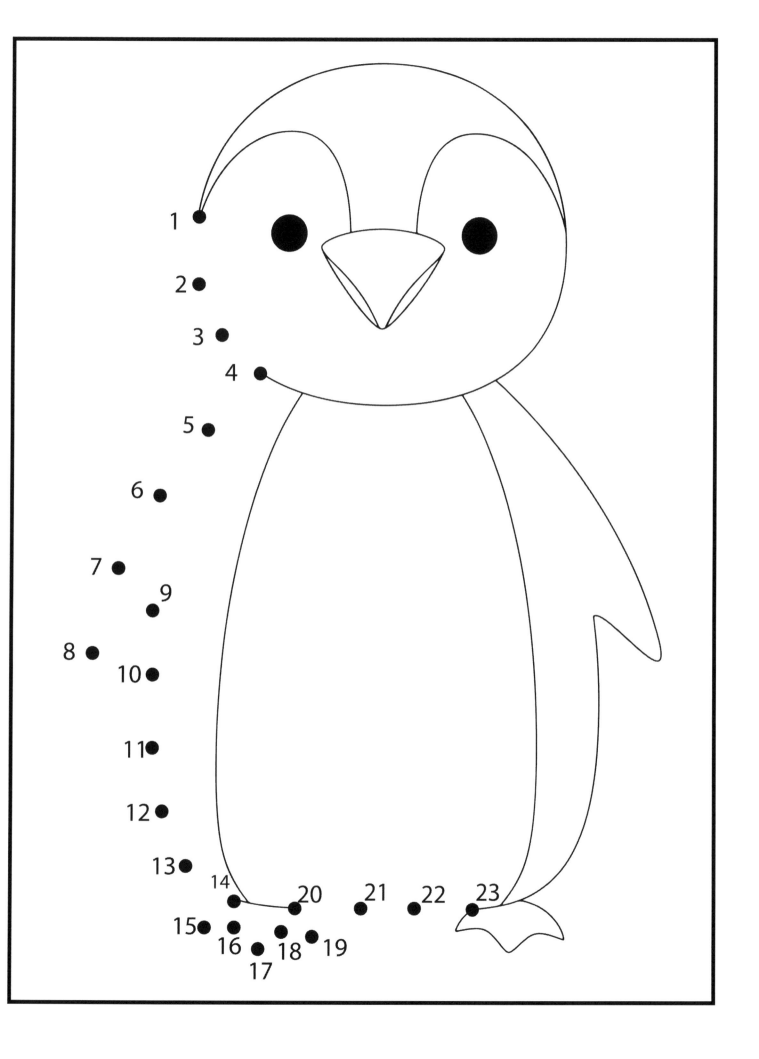

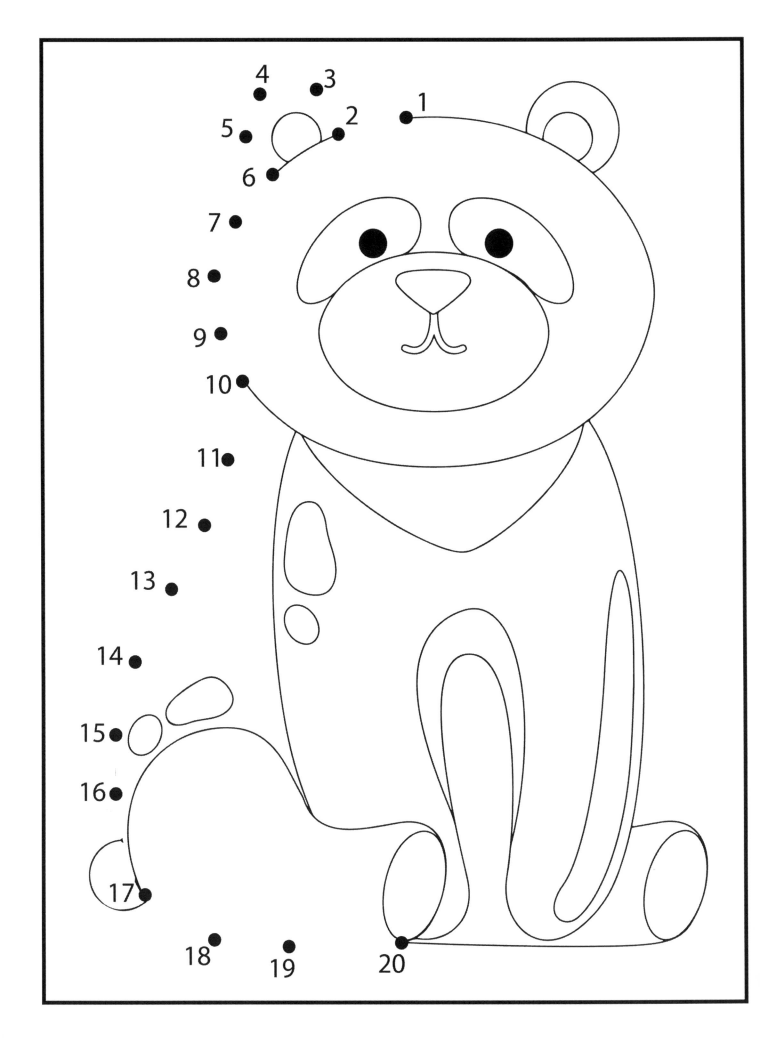

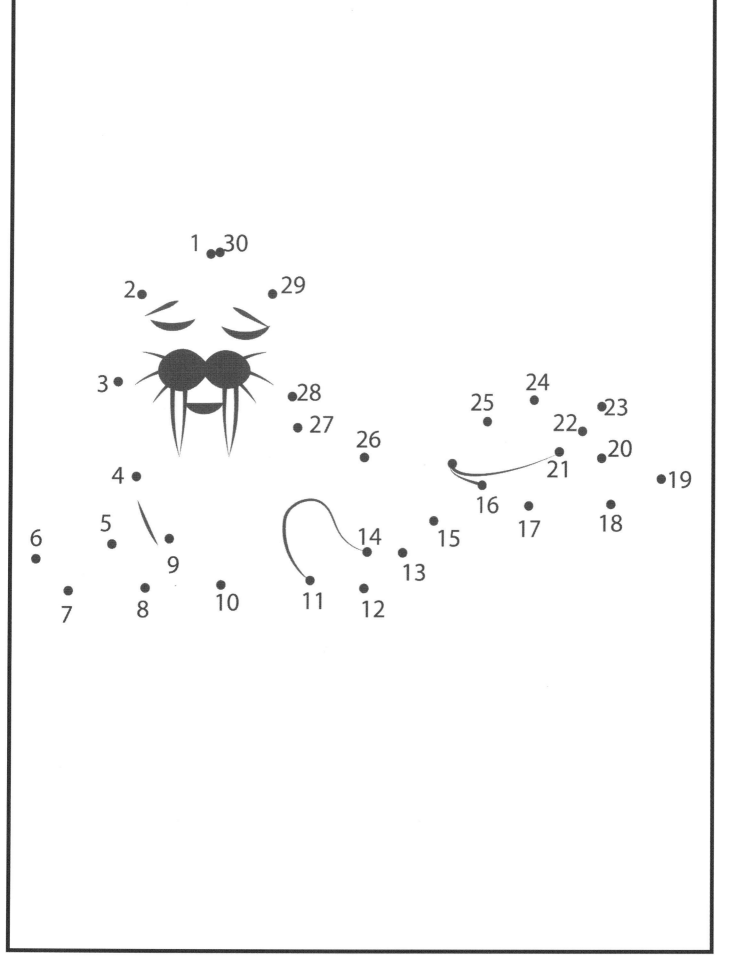

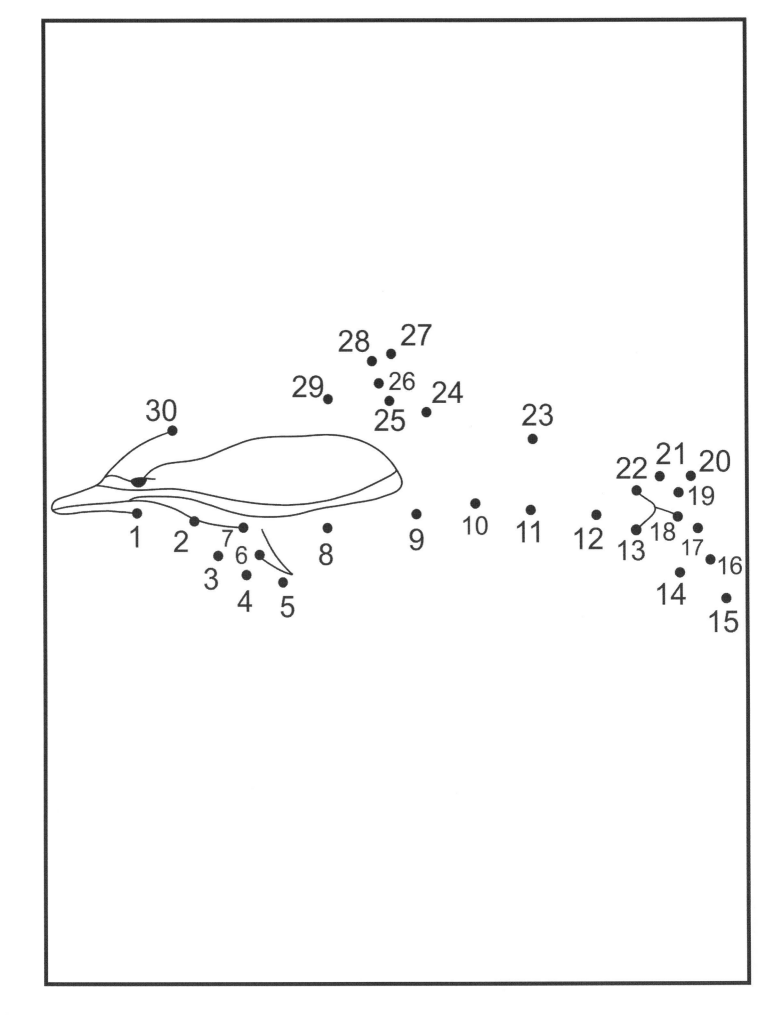

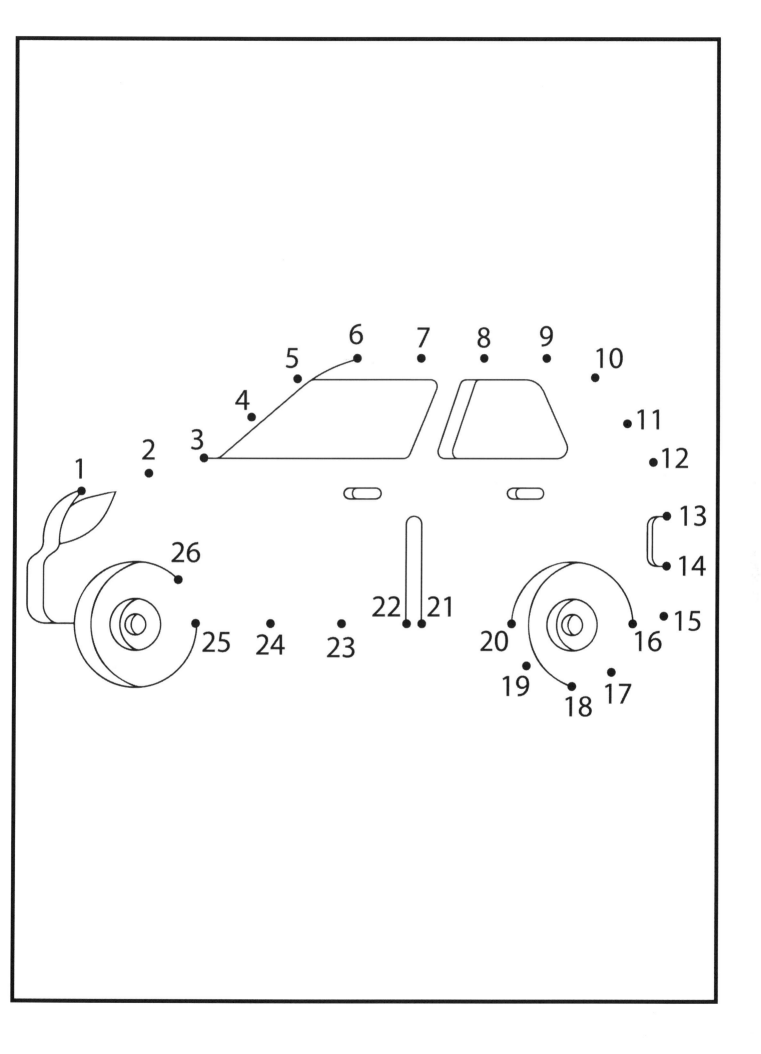

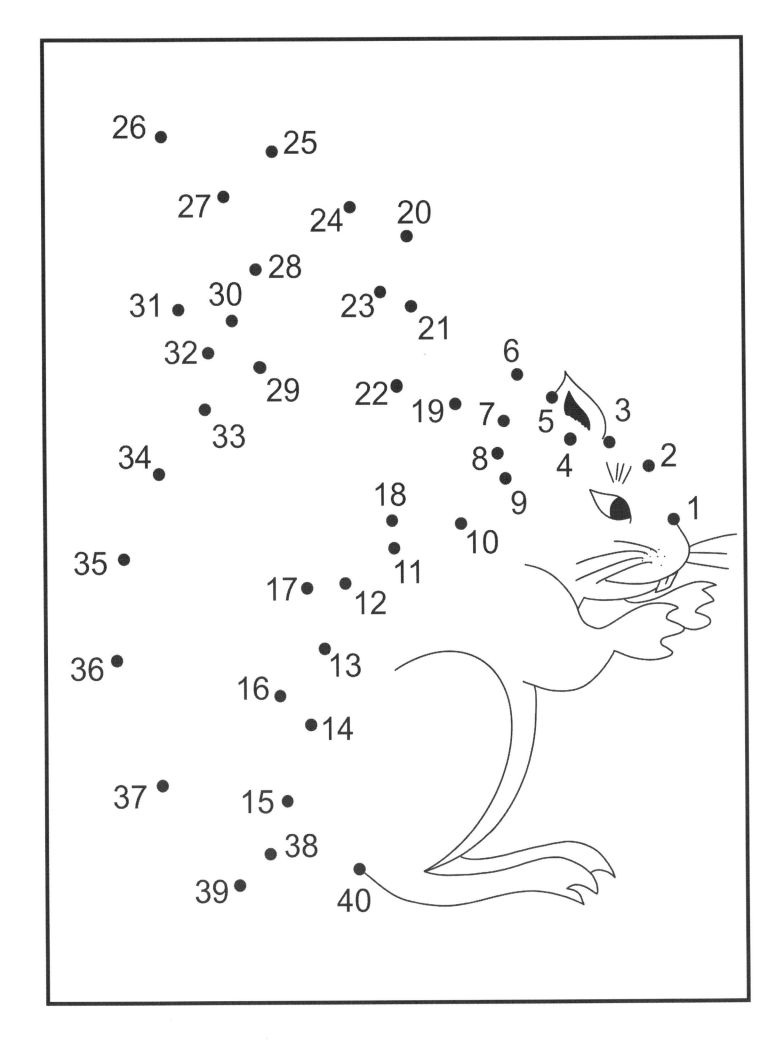

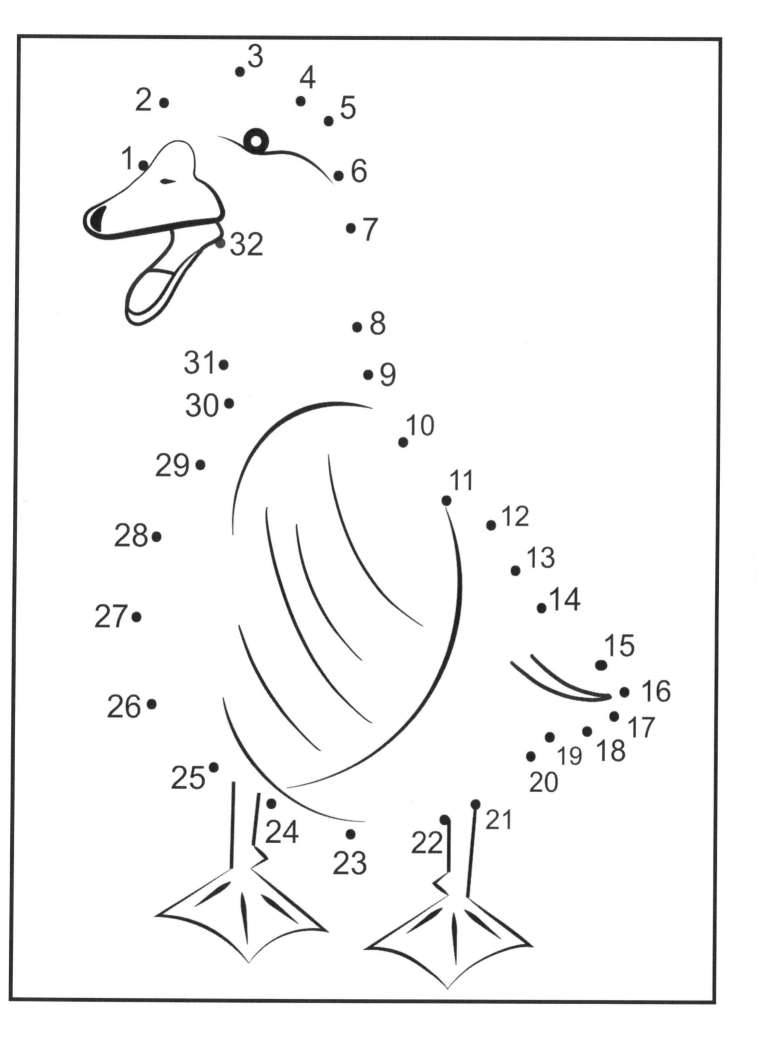

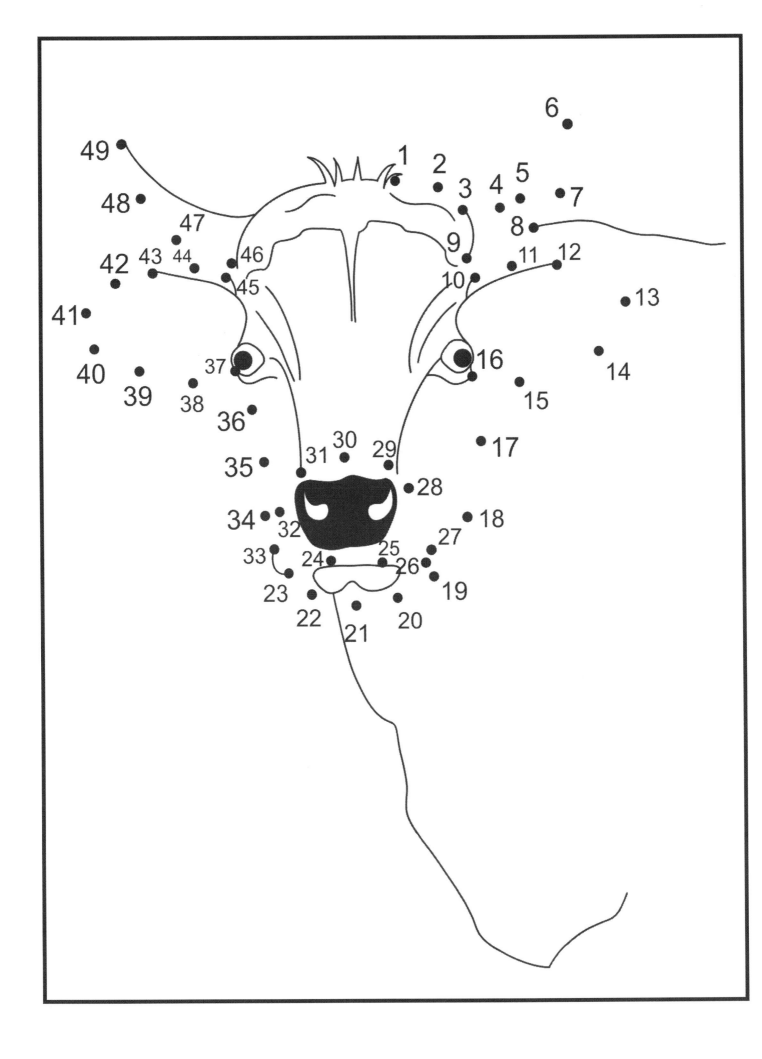

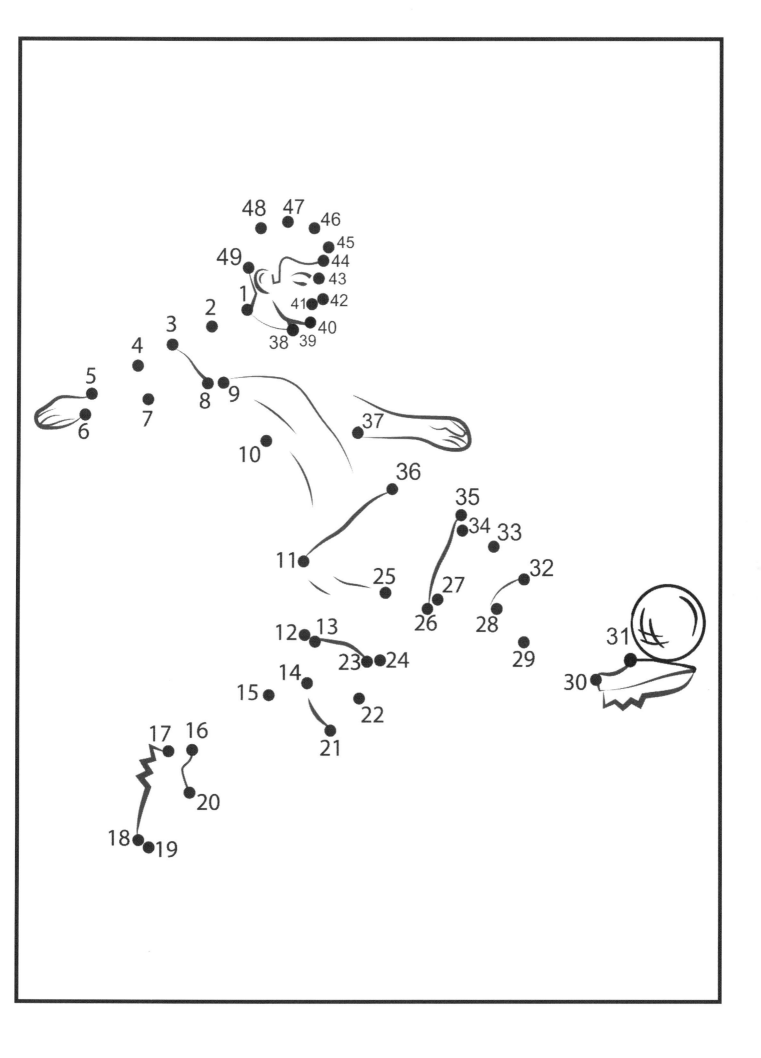

Made in United States
Orlando, FL
26 September 2024

51999896R00043